INTERNATIONAL CONGRESS AND SYMPOSIUM SERIES NUMBER 168

Editor-in-Chief: **Lord Walton of Detchant**

Aspirin—towards 2000

Proceedings of an international meeting sponsored by the European Aspirin Foundation, held in Brussels on 2–3 May, 1989

Edited by
Gordon Fryers

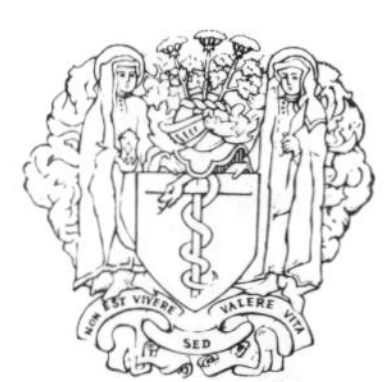

ROYAL SOCIETY OF MEDICINE SERVICES
LONDON · NEW YORK
1990

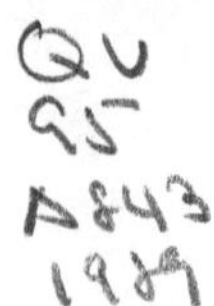

Royal Society of Medicine Services Limited
1 Wimpole Street London W1M 8AE
7 East 60th Street New York NY 10022

These proceedings are published by Royal Society of Medicine Services Ltd with financial support from the sponsor. The contributors are responsible for the scientific content and for the views expressed, which are not necessarily those of the sponsor, of the editor of the series or of the volume, of the Royal Society of Medicine or of Royal Society of Medicine Services Ltd. Distribution has been in accordance with the wishes of the sponsor but a copy is available to any Fellow of the Society at a privileged price.

British Library Cataloguing in Publication Data

Aspirin—towards 2000.
1. Medicine. Drug therapy. Aspirin
I. Fryers, G. R. (Gordon Robert) *1922–* II. Series
615.783

ISBN 1-85315-136-X

Phototypeset by Dobbie Typesetting Service, Tavistock, Devon
Printed in Great Britain at the Alden Press, Oxford

Participants

John Baum	*Professor of Medicine, Physical & Rehabilitation Medicine, School of Medicine & Dentistry, University of Rochester, New York, USA*
Fiona Broughton-Pipkin	*Reader in Reproductive Physiology, Department of Obstetrics and Gynaecology, Nottingham, UK*
Edward Cotlier	*Professor of Ophthalmology, King Saud University, Riyadh, Saudi Arabia*
Paul Davies	*Neurology Registrar, Department of Neurology, Charing Cross Hospital, London, UK*
Priscille Divry	*Department of Biochemistry, Hôpital Debrousse, Lyon, France*
Peter Evans	*Director of the Pain Clinic, Charing Cross Hospital, London, UK*
Frederick Frietag	*Assistant Director of the Diamond Headache Clinic, Chicago, USA*
Gordon Fryers ***(Editor & Session Chairman)***	*President of the European Aspirin Foundation, London, UK*
Giovanni De Gaetano	*Director of the Consorzio Mario, Negri Sud, Santa Maria Imbaro, Italy*
John Glasgow ***(Session Chairman)***	*Consultant Paediatrician, Reader in Child Health, The Queen's University of Belfast, Northern Ireland*
Allan L. Goldstein ***(Session Chairman)***	*Professor and Chairman of Department of Biochemistry & Molecular Biology, George Washington University Medical Centre, Washington DC, USA*
John Harding	*Senior Research Scientist, Nuffield Laboratory of Ophthalmology, Oxford, UK*

Jules Harris	*Samuel G Taylor III Professor of Medicine Director of the Rush Cancer Centre, Chicago, USA*
D. N. S. Kerr	*Dean of the Post Graduate Medical School, London, UK*
Alexander Mowat	*Consultant Paediatrician, Department of Child Health, King's College Hospital, London, UK*
Paolo Pozzilli	*Senior Lecturer, Department of Diabetics, Hotel-Dieu Hospital, Paris, France*
Clifford Rose **(Session Chairman)**	*Director of the Academic Unit of Neurosciences, Charing Cross & Westminster Medical School, London, UK*
Peter Sandercock	*Senior Lecturer, Department of Clinical Neuroscience, Western General Hospital, Edinburgh, Scotland, UK*
Gerard Slama	*Senior Lecturer, Department of Diabetics, Hotel-Dieu Hospital, Paris, France*
Bernard Spitz	*Assistant Professor, Department of Obstetrics and Gynaecology, University of Leuven, Belgium*
Michael de Swiet	*Consultant Physician, Queen Charlotte's Hospital, London, UK*
Serge Uzan	*Senior Lecturer, Head of Department of Obstetrics, Hôpital de l'Assistance Publique Tenon, Paris, France*
Joseph Vermylen **(Session Chairman)**	*Professor of Medicine, Centre for Thrombosis and Vascular Research, University of Leuven, Belgium*
Henk C. S. Wallenburg	*Professor of Obstetrics and Gynaecology, Head of Obstetrics Erasmus University Medical School, Rotterdam, The Netherlands*
Jerzy Wasserman	*Associate Professor & Director of the Central Microbiology Laboratory, The Karolinska Institute, Stockholm, Sweden*

Contents

The evidence concerning the role of eicosanoids in hypertensive pregnancy

Fiona Broughton-Pipkin

Department of Obstetrics and Gynaecology, University of Nottingham, UK

INTRODUCTION

Pregnancy-induced hypertension (PIH) is the occurrence of a blood pressure >140/90 mmHg on at least two separate occasions >24 h apart after the 20th week of pregnancy, in a woman known to be normotensive before this time and in whom the blood pressure has returned to normality by the 6th post-partum week. A diastolic blood pressure >120 mmHg constitutes severe PIH, and indeed many would regard a diastolic blood pressure of >110 mmHg as indicating the severe form of the disease. If proteinuria of >500 mg/24 h urine sample is also present, the condition is known as pre-eclampsia.

This is primarily a disease of first pregnancy, and in such women it occurs in a mild late-onset form in up to 20% of all primigravidae. This is a very high proportion and it poses the question whether it represents the high limit of the spectrum of normality, so that this mild, late-onset form is not a disease but a physiological process. This is borne out by the fact that the perinatal mortality and morbidity are no worse than those of the normotensive population. Also, the birth weight of the infants is certainly no worse and, in some studies, was shown to be slightly greater than that of the normotensive population.

However, the earlier the hypertension occurs, the more severe does the condition become, particularly when it is accompanied by proteinuria. It is characterized by increasing perinatal mortality and morbidity, decreasing birth weight, increasing maternal morbidity and—in the worst cases—mortality. In the most recent report on the *Confidential Inquiry into Maternal Deaths in the United Kingdom*, hypertensive disease was the single factor most frequently cited in association with maternal death. This is so in almost all the countries of western Europe where accurate records are kept, and in countries like those of central America and black Africa the problem becomes considerably worse. It is a major problem in many parts of the world.

We are hindered in our studies of this condition because no naturally-occurring animal model is yet known. Whether this relates to a haemodynamic or an anatomical difference related to our bipedal stance we do not know, but it markedly limits the opportunities for research. In the study of any disease process the early stages of its development are very important, but to study this in humans has proved to be extremely difficult.

Aspirin—towards 2000, edited by G. R. Fryers, 1990; Royal Society of Medicine Services International Congress and Symposium Series No. 168, published by Royal Society of Medicine Services Limited.

THEORETICAL BASIS FOR PREGNANCY-INDUCED HYPERTENSION

Two features have so far been identified which antedate the clinically apparent disease: first, there is an inadequate secondary trophoblast invasion and secondly there is an enhanced pressor response to angiotensin II.

In a normal pregnancy there is an invasion of trophoblast, that is, tissue of embryonic rather than maternal origin, which invades the walls of the spiral arteries. It erodes the muscular elastic tissue, so that what would normally be a reactive artery is actually converted into a conduit with floppy walls. However, in hypertensive pregnancy, this secondary wave of trophoblast invasion is halted at the deciduo-myometrial junction so that, proximal to that, the vessel is left in a reactive state capable of responding to hormonal and nervous stimuli.

We do not yet know what causes this halt, but we do think that the eicosanoids are involved because otherwise, in a normal or abnormal pregnancy, one would expect activation of the various clotting systems and fibrin deposition following the endothelial damage and erosion of these walls.

Arachidonic acid is a fatty acid which acts as a substrate for two important enzyme systems; lipoxygenase and cyclo-oxygenase, but I will concentrate on the cyclo-oxygenase side of the cascade. Under the action of this enzyme, arachidonic acid is converted into cyclic endoperoxides which are then further converted into various eicosanoids, prostacyclin, thromboxane, and the prostaglandins, particularly those of the E and F series.

Prostacyclin PGI_2 is a hormone predominantly produced in the walls of the arterial vasculature and it has two primary actions; it is a very potent vasodilator, relaxing vascular smooth muscle, and it inhibits platelet aggregation. The thromboxane (TxA_2) pathway directly counterbalances this: thromboxane is primarily produced by platelets and is pro-aggregatory and powerfully vasoconstrictive. It is not a circulating hormone and prostacyclin is probably not either; they are locally generated and locally active. Endothelial damage normally activates the thromboxane pathway, but obviously this is not happening when the spiral arteries are being eroded.

PGI_2 synthesis increases markedly in normal pregnancy, as assessed from concentrations of its urinary metabolites. However, women who suffer the more severe form of PIH show reduced excretion of prostacyclin metabolite from the start of pregnancy, well before hypertension is apparent. This result must be treated with caution, because the kidneys themselves can produce high concentrations of the vasodilator prostanoids, so that this diminution might only reflect decreased renal production, but still it is suggestive. The balance between PGI_2:TxA_2 would thus be shifted towards vasoconstriction and platelet aggregation.

The other feature that antedates the onset of PIH is a change in pressor response to angiotensin II. In normotension outside pregnancy, the plasma concentration of circulating angiotensin II is just below that which could affect blood pressure. In normal pregnancy, this concentration increases as a response to salt loss caused by progesterone. However, there is protection against the potential pressor effects of this so that much more angiotensin II is needed in pregnancy to get the same rise in pressure. The eicosanoids are implicated in this. The E series eicosanoids and angiotensin II counterbalance each other, and angiotensin II also stimulates the production of vasodilator eicosanoids, which themselves in turn stimulate increased renin release. Renin is a necessary precursor for the production of angiotensin II, so they are mutually supporting.

It has been known for more than 20 years that in hypertensive pregnancy, this protection is lost. Normotensive pregnant women need increasing amounts of angiotensin II to evoke a given rise in blood pressure in the first trimester, then it stabilizes and in the last few weeks of pregnancy the responsiveness starts to return to non-pregnant values. However, in women who subsequently become hypertensive, pressor sensitivity returns towards non-pregnant values much earlier. They become more sensitive.

One reason for this might be the inadequate production of vasodilator eicosanoids, which in fact occurs. The concentrations of eicosanoids in tissues arising from hypertensives differ from those arising from normotensive pregnant women. The concentration of prostacyclin metabolites is reduced among hypertensives in tissue and in the plasma of both uterine and peripheral venous circulations. Where the generation of thromboxane or its metabolites has been measured, concentrations are shown to be either unchanged or perhaps slightly greater, but even so the balance between prostacyclin and thromboxane has shifted towards the vasoconstrictor pro-aggregatory side.

EXPERIMENTAL EVIDENCE

As the prostanoids are normally involved in decreasing pressor responsiveness to angiotensin II, the effects can be mimicked in an animal situation. Some years ago, we examined in pregnant rabbits the effects of the direct administration of vasodilator prostanoids on the pressor response to angiotensin II. We found a rightward parallel shift of the dose-response curve with increasing doses of prostaglandin E_2. Other similar experiments, which involved decreasing circulating vasodilatory eicosanoid concentrations, showed an enhanced response to angiotensin II. Pregnant rabbits fed a diet as nearly as possible totally deficient in essential fatty acids, developed an increased pressor response to angiotensin II. Thus, deficiency of the predominantly vasodilatory prostanoids resulted in an increased pressor response; addition of the vasodilatory prostanoids decreased the pressor response.

The experimental emphasis then moved to humans, with all the human experiments being done in women whose pregnancies were to be terminated in the second trimester on social grounds, so that their pregnancies were not in fact continuing, even though they were physiologically normal at the time of experiment. Repeating the animal experiments achieved similar results; the presence of a vasodilator prostaglandin at a dose insufficient to affect the basal blood pressure lowered the pressor response to angiotensin II.

Does increasing the endogenous production of vasodilator prostanoids have an effect on angiotensin II response? Evening primrose oil contains the precursors for the PGE_1 series, which are vasodilatory. We asked women entering hospital for termination of pregnancy to ingest a high dose of evening primrose oil for a week beforehand. We then infused angiotensin II and found that in all cases the response was less than the mean response for an unsupplemented group as a whole. This difference was statistically highly significant.

If renal blood flow is reduced, the kidney responds by synthesizing increased amounts of renin which act on its substrate producing angiotensin I, which is converted in the kidneys and pulmonary circulation to angiotensin II. This angiotensin II increases the systemic blood pressure, but in the kidney it acts to promote the synthesis of the vasodilators prostacyclin and PGE_2. The overall effect is that, although systemic blood pressure rises, renal perfusion is improved.

The kidneys are a very important organ and this mechanism is powerful enough to override the sympathetic nervous system and all the normal controls for the blood pressure.

In pregnancies which become hypertensive, and in those too which suffer from intra-uterine growth retardation (IUGR), there is a failure of the secondary wave of trophoblast invasion. This will have the effect of cutting down the blood flow once the foetal demands for oxygen and nutrients exceed a certain level. It does not matter in early pregnancy, but at some stage in late pregnancy it will matter and a degree of worsening ischaemia in the foeto-placental unit will ensue. There is some evidence that this has precisely the same effects as ischaemia in the kidney: that the ischaemic foeto-placental unit synthesizes renin and releases it into the systemic circulation. Paired measurements of peripheral and uterine venous blood at caesarean section show that there is indeed an increased release of renin and angiotensin II into the systemic circulation in pregnancies complicated by hypertension.

Data have been obtained comparing the *in vitro* basal production of the prostacyclin metabolite 6-keto-$F_{1\alpha}$ by non-pregnant, pregnant, early post-partum and late post-partum tissues from the uterine arteries and the omental arteries. In a normal pregnancy the uterine arteries synthesize large amounts of prostacyclin. As prostacyclin production is stimulated by angiotensin II, there is the possibility of the same kind of inter-relationship in a mildly hypertensive pregnancy. We know that the sympathetic nervous system is not involved in mild PIH; indeed, it appears to be down-regulated.

If the woman cannot produce the eicosanoids there will be increased production of the potent vasoconstrictor angiotensin II and an increase in systemic arterial pressure so, if the foeto-placental unit cannot synthesize sufficient prostacyclin, then matters deteriorate. This could also explain the breakdown in renal function because, again, a common failure of prostacyclin production in the renal circulation will cause the renal circulation to shut down. In the severe forms of PIH that is exactly what happens.

CONCLUSION

The mild form of pregnancy-induced hypertension may, in fact, not be pathological and should not be treated as such. It is an example of the foetus with its own needs for the survival of the species overriding the temporary needs of the mother. Once that foetus and placenta are delivered, the mother's blood pressure returns to normal. It appears that it is only when a vital part of this compensatory physiological control mechanism breaks down that the severe, potentially life-threatening hypertension, renal failure and widely-disseminated intravascular coagulation supervene.

The effects of aspirin therapy on vascular reactivity and prostaglandin metabolism

Bernard Spitz

Department of Obstetrics and Gynaecology, University of Leuven, Belgium

Gestational proteinuric hypertension may be associated with an imbalance between prostacyclin and thromboxane—eicosanoids with potent and opposing effects on vascular reactivity—and platelet aggregation. The normal pregnant woman becomes refractory to the effect of angiotensin II and more of the substance is needed to increase systolic blood pressure; women who will develop gestational hypertension begin losing angiotensin II refractoriness as early as 18 weeks of pregnancy, before clinical symptoms become apparent.

There is evidence that various haemodynamic changes characteristic of normal pregnancy may depend on the balance between production of vasodilator and vasoconstrictor eicosanoids, and that prostacyclin and thromboxane could be involved in this phenomenon. Animal evidence supports this contention, but if pregnant rats are dosed with aspirin on day 14, they react like non-pregnant animals again. When prostacyclin is given to pregnant rats without affecting baseline blood pressure it makes them mimic pregnant ones. Whereas normal pregnancy may be characterized by increasing prostacyclin production, relative to thromboxane, in pregnancy-induced hypertension (PIH) the production of these two eicosanoids appears to be tilted towards thromboxane.

Enhanced sensitivity to the pressor effects of angiotensin II could be an early sign of such an imbalance. The beneficial effects of low dose aspirin in preventing PIH have been attributed to the suppression of thromboxane synthesis, with a sparing of prostacyclin. The cyclo-oxygenase of platelets could be more sensitive or prone to irreversible acetylation by aspirin and anuclear platelets and, in contrast to endothelial cells, for instance, cannot synthesize new enzyme.

LOW-DOSE ASPIRIN AND VASCULAR REACTIVITY

The aim of our study was to determine the effects of low-dose aspirin on changes in vascular reactivity due to angiotensin II, and to see if a change in vascular reactivity could be explained by alterations in circulating prostacyclin and thromboxane. Therefore, we performed angiotensin II sensitivity tests in an at-risk population. The women were placed in a quiet room in the left lateral position; blood pressure and heart rate were measured every four minutes using an automatic oscillometric method. After stabilization of diastolic blood pressure,

Aspirin—towards 2000, edited by G. R. Fryers, 1990; Royal Society of Medicine Services International Congress and Symposium Series No. 168, published by Royal Society of Medicine Services Limited.

an intravenous infusion of angiotensin II was initiated and gradually increased. The test was stopped after the effective pressor dose, which is the minimum amount of angiotensin II required to increase diastolic blood pressure by 20 mmHg, was determined in duplicate. Before the infusion of angiotensin II, urine and blood was collected for analysis of angiotensin II and prostaglandin metabolites.

We obtained a group of 25 non-sensitive and one of 22 sensitive women. In the angiotensin II-sensitive women, namely those with an effective pressor dose of <10 ng/kg/min, the test and analysis of metabolites was repeated after one week's treatment with aspirin 81 mg daily, which is just one-quarter of a grain.

There was no significant difference in weight, age, systolic or diastolic blood pressure, or gestational age between the non-sensitive and sensitive groups.

A surprising finding was that, for equal blood pressures, the baseline heart rate was significantly slower in the sensitive group. It seems that the sensitive women, faced with increased peripheral resistance, initially tried to maintain a normal blood pressure by decreasing their heart rate. This mechanism could also contribute to the decrease in utero-placental flow, and simply measuring pulse rate in pregnant women seems to us a useful screening test. We could detect approximately 50% of women who were going to develop gestational hypertension just by measuring pulse rate at 28 weeks.

The decrease in heart rate while the effective pressor dose was given, a measure of baroreceptor function, was not different between the non-sensitive and sensitive groups. These data do not support reports that baroreceptor function is lost in early pre-eclampsia and is responsible for the instability of the blood pressure and the sensitivity to vasopressors.

It is interesting to note that although sensitive and non-sensitive women were clinically indistinguishable apart from the pulse rate, urinary 2,3,dinorthromboxane metabolites in angiotensin II-sensitive women were already significantly higher than in normal, non-sensitive ones. After one week's aspirin treatment, the effective pressor dose in the angiotensin II-sensitive group overall rose from 5.9 ± 2.4 ($X \pm SD$) to 10.2 ± 5.5 ng/kg/min ($p<0.01$), demonstrating that the treatment does indeed decrease vascular sensitivity. Platelet-derived serum thromboxane B_2, a stable metabolite of thromboxane A_2, a measure for compliance with therapy, decreased from 1804 ± 1771 to 132 ± 206 pg/ml ($p<0.01$). Plasma thromboxane B_2 also decreased from 130 ± 107 to 19 ± 12 pg/ml ($p<0.01$). Although there was an overall significant improvement, about half of the women remained sensitive and eventually developed clinical disease, despite maintaining the aspirin intake. As expected, the improvement in the sensitive group after aspirin treatment could not be explained by a change in cardiac response.

After one week of aspirin treatment, thromboxane formation is proportionally more inhibited (86%) than the production of either prostacyclin or prostaglandin E_2, both of which were inhibited by 30–40%. The prostacyclin/thromboxane ratio rose from about 3.1 ± 2.0 before aspirin treatment to 12.4 ± 9.9 ($p<0.01$) after treatment. In other studies, normal pregnant women required a similar effective pressor dose, about 20 ng/kg/min, and after non-selective inhibition by high-dose aspirin or indomethacin, decreased to more or less the same 'non-pregnant' intermediate values.

We believe that oral inhibition by means of aspirin 81 mg daily was non-selective, at least in nulliparous women, for there could be a difference between nulli- and multiparous women. Absolute prostacyclin formation was affected and decrease of plasma 6-keto-$PGF_{1\alpha}$, which reached 30% in our study, could represent a more dramatic feature at the level of the vessel wall.

Aspirin, 1 mg/kg/day, which is approximately the dose used in the Collaborative Study of Low Dose Aspirin in Pregnancy (CLASP), had a significant effect on prostacyclin production by the vessels in rats. It was administered intramuscularly, which might make a difference, and of course murine metabolism might not be the same, but a dose as low as the equivalent of about 20 mg/day had a less pronounced, but still pronounced effect on prostacyclin production by vessels.

CONCLUSIONS

If normal pregnancy is characterized by prostacyclin, and pre-eclampsia by thromboxane dominance, then non-selective prostacyclin inhibition will increase effective pressor dose in pre-eclamptic women and decrease it in normal pregnant women, to the same neutral, intermediate non-pregnant level. It is conceivable that, by preventing thromboxane domination, even non-selective prostacyclin inhibition could reduce the incidence or severity of PIH, but elimination of the condition is unlikely to be achieved.

The collaborative study of low-dose aspirin in pregnancy

Michael de Swiet

Queen Charlotte's Hospital, London, UK

INTRODUCTION

CLASP stands for Collaborative Low-dose Aspirin Study in Pregnancy, and it is very much a collaborative study. Initially it was planned as a collaborative study in the UK only, but there has been considerable interest worldwide and so it has now been extended to become truly international. The study is funded for a total of three years, primarily by the Medical Research Council in the United Kingdom, but also from other supporting agencies such as the Aspirin Foundation.

Pre-eclampsia affects 10–20% of all pregnancies; it is a major cause of maternal death, probably the most common cause of iatrogenic prematurity or induction at term, certainly a common cause of growth retardation, may cause problems with the baby in delivery, and really it is only the delivery that modifies its effects. It is perhaps the reason for half of ante-natal care in the latter half of pregnancy.

BACKGROUND TO CLASP

Our starting points were the clinical trials of Beaufils and Uzan (1), that of Wallenburg (2), and more recently a trial published by Brian Trudinger in Australia (3). Wallenburg (2) studied low-dose aspirin vs placebo in a group of women shown to be at risk of developing pre-eclampsia. The results were very convincing, but the study was small and the conditions really not applicable to clinical practice. Uzan's (1) study was more applicable to clinical practice because patients were chosen on clinical criteria, but that preliminary trial was not really large enough to detect important side-effects. An interesting study was done by the Australian obstetrician Trudinger (3), who was looking primarily at intrauterine growth retardation (IUGR) rather than pre-eclampsia, although the two may share a common pathology. His results indicated that low-dose aspirin could possibly reduce IUGR. He selected pregnancies where the baby was thought to be at rsk of IUGR because of abnormal flow patterns in the umbilical blood vessels, as detected ultrasonically. Those babies whose mothers were given low-dose aspirin were about 500 g larger in size at birth than those born to untreated mothers.

These were our starting points, plus our own clinical experience. We reviewed the pregnancies we had managed with aspirin at Queen Charlotte's and

Aspirin—towards 2000, edited by G. R. Fryers, 1990; Royal Society of Medicine Services International Congress and Symposium Series No. 168, published by Royal Society of Medicine Services Limited.

Hammersmith Hospitals in London, and compared them with previous pregnancies. In the previous, high-risk pregnancy, there was only a 10% live birth rate. When we treated the women with aspirin there was an 87% live birth rate. Our study was uncontrolled, so the circumstances of management in the second pregnancy might have been better than the circumstances in the first pregnancy, but the results were certainly persuasive.

POSSIBILITIES OF ADVERSE EFFECTS

I believe it is quite likely that aspirin is effective, but I certainly do not think that we yet have sufficient data to prove overall efficacy, nor to be aware of possible side-effects which might be rare, occurring at the 1% level, but still important. It is, thus, important to review the possibilities of adverse effects in terms of teratogenesis, the effect on the foetal circulation, the foetal lung, inhibition of labour, blood clotting and Reye's syndrome.

Teratogenesis is, to a certain extent, not a problem. In the context of our clinical trial teratogenesis is unlikely, because we are starting treatment after 12 weeks of gestation, by which time the baby is more or less fully formed. It is, therefore, unlikely that aspirin could affect organs which have already been formed. A review of the literature provides a little evidence that there might be a problem, but it is by no means strong: two papers from the USA, one suggesting an increased risk of abnormality in the baby's feet (4) and the other a slightly increased risk of congenital heart disease (5). None of the cardiovascular abnormalities were significant when looked at alone, and they only achieved significance when the data were pooled—not a sensible thing to do on an embryological basis. The most compelling evidence of all came from a study in the USA involving 14 000 babies exposed to aspirin in early pregnancy, which could not detect any increased risk of teratogenesis (6). I would again emphasize that, in CLASP, the drug is being used after the time when teratogenesis might be expected.

The question of foetal circulation must also be addressed. It is extremely important that the ductus arteriosus, which links the two sides of foetal circulation, should remain open in intrauterine life. Its patency is maintained by prostaglandins (7) and it is possible that inhibition of prostaglandin synthesis by aspirin might cause closure of the ductus arteriosus, with subsequent circulatory problems. Indeed, there have been isolated case reports of this in the use of the much more highly active prostaglandin antagonist, indomethacin (7). However, there have been trials of indomethacin for use in pre-term labour showing no association between indomethacin and circulatory problems in the foetus (8). A large American study looked at babies exposed to aspirin later on in foetal life. After examining 26 000 mothers taking aspirin and comparing them to 15 000 controls, they found no increased risk of circulatory problems in the babies (9). So, although it is something to be aware of, it is probably not a major factor.

The question of abnormalities in the foetal lung being caused by suppression of prostaglandin synthesis is entirely theoretical and comes from giving much larger amounts of aspirin to experimental animals (7). Certainly the collaborative study mentioned above would not support the likelihood of damage to the foetal lung from aspirin.

It is quite possible that prostaglandins have some part to play in the mechanism of labour, so interfering with their synthesis might cause labour either to start later or to be more prolonged. The only way of finding out whether that is the case is by clinical trial of the sort that we are performing. The evidence that might suggest an action of aspirin in this way comes from studies done in Australia (10), where some of the women were essentially aspirin addicts and had been taking several grams of aspirin a day. Under those circumstances they did deliver their babies about a week later than did other controls, but it is quite possible that the other controls all had pre-eclampsia and needed to be induced earlier. Certainly the paper that describes this abnormality makes no comment on the difference between spontaneous and induced labour in this group of patients (10).

The question of blood clotting is, of course, absolutely inherent in the action of aspirin. If aspirin is working in the way we believe, it interferes with the aggregation of platelets, and so we need to be aware of a possible risk of bleeding, both in mothers and in their babies (11). Again, in the Australian study mentioned above (10), if the mothers were taking very large amounts of aspirin there was an increased risk of both post-partum haemorrhage and ante-partum haemorrhage. However, I would emphasize that these women were taking several grams of aspirin each day, as opposed to the 60 mg/day that we are considering. If the aspirin was taken within a few days of delivery, then the foetus was also at risk of bleeding and presumably the foetal platelets were inhibited in the same way as the maternal platelets would have been. But again, one must be aware of the very large dosages involved, compared to those which are being used in CLASP.

Reye's syndrome is associated with a febrile illness, so we think it is unlikely that our newborn babies are going to be affected by the condition. Again there is a question of dose; the usual dose in children who develop Reye's syndrome is 10 mg/kg (12), while we are only administering 10% of that, even if all the aspirin were distributed evenly within the foetus, which is an exceedingly unlikely event. The median age of presentation of Reye's syndrome is also far later, about 14 months of age (12), and neonatal Reye's syndrome is almost unheard of. If it does occur it is probably a congenital abnormality of metabolism such that the baby cannot handle various substances normally.

After deciding that the risk of adverse effects was very small, and in the knowledge that considerable amounts of aspirin have been administered during pregnancy, either advertently or inadvertently, we are reasonably confident in going ahead with a clinical trial.

METHODOLOGY

There are two possible ways to construct a trial for this particular problem. One could either have fixed entry criteria, being very precise in the sorts of patient recruited, or one could allow a flexible entry approach. If you have fixed entry criteria, you certainly know exactly the sort of patients entering your trial group: they will be those who have suffered a precise degree of hypertension, or a precise degree of growth retardation, in a previous pregnancy. Inevitably, if you instil such precision, the number of patients you recruit will be exceedingly restricted. The statistics are very easy because you have one simple trial group compared to one simple placebo group, but statistical methods are now sophisticated enough to allow much more complicated analyses depending on stratification, a comparison of the severely affected patients in the trial group with the severely affected patients in the placebo group. The problem with such fixed entry criteria is that they only answer one question, the question of what aspirin might do in people who presented with a certain blood pressure level in the past. More importantly this form of trial does not test clinical practice as it occurs.

Although on the basis of such a trial we could define patients who might or might not be improved on the basis of aspirin therapy, clinical practice is not like that. Physicians base their judgments on many factors including their own experience, so we have chosen a very flexible trial which will test clinical practice as it actually is, or will become. This makes it easier to select patients; inevitably the trial will have to be larger, but one can perform stratification at entry and certainly at the time of analysis and this allows several questions to be answered.

The fundamental entry criterion is that the clinician should be uncertain whether or not aspirin will help this patient who has suffered pre-eclampsia or IUGR in the past, or who may be developing these conditions in the index pregnancy. If the clinician believes that the condition is so mild that aspirin therapy is unnecessary, it would be unethical to randomize the patient to aspirin or placebo. Conversely, if the clinician believes the circumstances to be so severe that the patient must be given aspirin, it might be considered unethical to withhold aspirin. However, in the majority of cases, there will be an element of uncertainty and that is the criterion of entry to the trial.

AIMS OF THE CLASP STUDY

We believe we will need to recruit about 4000 patients in order to achieve results with 95% certainty. Perhaps the first aim is the most important: a reduction in proteinuric pre-eclampsia of 25%. If the reduction was only 5% it might be of biological interest but it would not be of much clinical significance, so we decided that this was the level of reduction of proteinuric pre-eclampsia that would be important to our colleagues. As a corollary to that, we would also expect to show, if it occurred, an increase in the corrected birthweight of at least 100 g, or an increase in maturity at the time of delivery of one day. An increase in maturity at the time of delivery of one day is not important in itself, but that comes as a consequence of the other criteria.

ENTRY CRITERIA

The eligibility criteria are essentially based on gestational age, between 12 and 32 weeks. Before 12 weeks, there are concerns about teratogenesis, and it is unlikely that aspirin is necessary as early in pregnancy because the placental abnormalities only become apparent at about 12–14 weeks. After 32 weeks' gestation, if there are problems with hypertension or IUGR in pregnancy, current thinking is that the baby is better delivered. If our study shows that the drug is helpful in these conditions it might be preferable to start aspirin therapy after 32 weeks, because it would generally be better to deliver at 37 weeks rather than 36 weeks, but in the present state of knowledge a 32-week cut-off is being maintained.

The indications for entry are either because of experience during a previous pregnancy in terms of hypertension or IUGR, or signs that such abnormalities might be occurring in this pregnancy. In terms of prophylaxis, we would consider previous high blood pressure or previous IUGR, and then other factors that might tip the balance in deciding whether or not such a person should be randomized. These might include such items as whether there is a past medical history of high blood pressure or diabetes, whether the woman is relatively old and so on.

From the point of view of therapeutic entry, again early signs of high blood pressure or IUGR will decide.

Exclusion criteria are first of all those who are going to be delivered very soon because their condition is so severe. It would be unwise to give aspirin when hypertension is so severe that delivery will probably be needed within a few days. Those with a high risk of bleeding, usually because of their past history or because they have bleeding tendencies, and those who have actually had a placental haemorrhage in previous pregnancies, will also be excluded. This is a group in whom aspirin might be helpful, but we are concerned that hypertension in pregnancy also increases the risk of placental haemorrhage, and aspirin might make the bleeding worse, so for the moment we would rather exclude such patients. Others excluded are those with aspirin allergy, and women suffering from asthma, which increases the risk of aspirin allergy. We have excluded patients with systemic lupus erythematosus from our trial because there is soon likely to be another major international study, looking at aspirin in that specific group of patients.

RECRUITMENT

The trial started at the beginning of January 1988, and by the end of October 1988 a large number of hospitals in the UK were involved, a total of 127 hospitals and 430 doctors. We consider that to be a remarkable achievement on the part of our scientific statistical group, who have been responsible for the administration of the trial, because that probably represents over half the doctors practising hospital obstetrics in the United Kingdom. Subsequently there has been international interest and doctors from a number of other countries are taking part in the study.

With regard to patient recruitment to the study, until the end of March 1989 we had recruited about 1100 patients. Of those in the prophylactic group, the majority have been recruited because of pre-eclampsia in previous pregnancies and a smaller number because of IUGR. The group treated therapeutically is much smaller, but again hypertension is the principal reason for treatment rather than IUGR.

REFERENCES

(1) Beaufils M, Uzan S. Prevention of pre-eclampsia by early antiplatelet therapy. *Lancet* 1985; **i**: 840–2.

(2) Wallenburg HCS, Makovitz JW. Low-dose aspirin prevents pregnancy-induced hypertension and pre-eclampsia in angiotensin-sensitive primigravidae. *Lancet* 1986; **i**: 1–3.

(3) Trudinger BJ, Cook CM, Thompson RS, Giles WB, Connelly A. Low-dose aspirin therapy improves fetal weight in umbilical placental insufficiency. *Am J Obstet Gynecol* 1988; **159**: 681–5.

(4) Richards ID. Congenital malformations and environmental influence in pregnancy. *Br J Prevent Soc Med* 1969; **23**: 218.

(5) Zierler S, Rothman KJ. Congenital heart disease in relation to maternal use of vendctin and other drugs in early pregnancy. *N Engl J Med* 1985; **313**: 347–52.

(6) Slone D, Siskino V, Heinonen OP, Monson RP, Kaufman DW. Aspirin and congenital malformations. *Lancet* 1976; **i**: 1373–5.

(7) Heymann MA. Non-steroidal anti-inflammatory agents. In: Eskes TKAB, Finster M, eds. *Drug therapy during pregnancy*. London: Butterworths, 1985: 85.

(8) Nierbyl JR, Blake DA, White RD, *et al.* The inhibition of premature labour with indomethacin. *Am J Obstet Gynec* 1980; **136**: 1014.
(9) Shapiro S, Siskino V, Monson R, Heinonen OP, Kaufman DW, Slone D. Perinatal mortality and birth-weight in relation to aspirin later during pregnancy. *Lancet* 1976; **i**: 1375–6.
(10) Collins E, Turner G. Maternal effects of regular salicylate ingestion in pregnancy. *Lancet* 1975; **ii**: 335–9.
(11) Stuart MJ, Gross SJ, Elrad H, Graeber JE. Effects of acetylsalicylic-acid ingestion on maternal and neonatal hemostasis. *N Engl J Med* 1982; **307**: 909–12.
(12) Notes and News. Reye's syndrome and the giving of aspirin to children. *Lancet* 1986; **i**: 1396.

DISCUSSION

Dr Cotlier: Many of the women at various times in pregnancy have headaches and other pains and sometimes they take aspirin. How is it possible to eliminate completely the isolated taking of aspirin by pregnant women during their pregnancy? Is that feasible or can you determine whether there have been any violations of your protocol?

Dr de Swiet: Clearly this is a problem we have considered. First, the patients are advised that if they have headaches or other pains they should not take aspirin but paracetamol, which is a mild and safe analgesic. Secondly, if despite that they do take aspirin, we have no reason to believe that the people in the placebo group are more likely to take aspirin than those in the treated group, so we are relying on the double-blind placebo-controlled nature of the trial to balance it out. We accept that there may be a weakening of the effect of aspirin because of illicit aspirin taking, or for that matter non-compliance, but we believe it is unlikely that this will give us artificially good results, rather giving us artificially bad results.

Dr Sandercock: Have women's groups been involved in the design and execution of this study and, if so, what is their attitude to randomization?

Dr de Swiet: Yes, they have been involved. They had some conceptual difficulties with randomization but, in the end, agreed to it. One of the problems that we found from the women's groups' point of view was that they would tend to look at pregnancy-induced hypertension from their immediate experience, usually the experience of their own pregnancies. Really severe hypertension in pregnancy can be a catastrophic event but it does not affect very many women and, for that reason, women's groups sometimes thought that we were just making a fuss about nothing. In the end, after full consultation, they are behind us.

Professor Wallenburg: In addition, some years ago we conducted a controlled study of the effect of low-dose aspirin in women with repeated severe foetal growth retardation (1,2). We designed it as a placebo-controlled trial, but the first 10 or so women refused, because they said: 'I don't know what aspirin does, but a dummy is a dummy and I am not going to take a dummy because I already lost two babies. If you want to try your aspirin on me, that's fine, but I am not going to take a dummy.' So we could not do the study in that highly selected group with a bad obstetric history.

Dr de Swiet: We have had the same problem but it works both ways. I have had patients who have said to me: 'Yes, I will only enter the trial if I can be certain I will get aspirin.' Yet I have had other patients who have said: 'I will only enter the trial if I can be certain that I will get placebo.' I do not mean to denigrate women, I really understand the difficulties they have.

REFERENCES

(1) Wallenburg HC, Rotmans N. Prevention of recurrent idiopathic fetal growth retardation by low-dose aspirin and dipyridamole. *Am J Obstet Gynecol* 1987; **157**: 1230–5.
(2) Trudinger B, Cook CM, Thompson R, Giles W, Connelly A. Low-dose aspirin improves fetal weight in umbilical placental insufficiency. (Letter) *Lancet* 1988; **ii**: 214–5.

Clinical trials of prevention of intra-uterine growth retardation with aspirin

Serge Uzan

Department of Obstetrics, Hôpital Tenon, Paris, France

INTRODUCTION

The treatment of intrauterine growth retardation (IUGR), with or without associated hypertension, and the complications of pregnancy-induced hypertension is most often purely palliative. Delivery of the foetus is usually the only choice, and this often results in serious prematurity and neonatal problems. Numerous studies have attempted to analyse the phenomena responsible for these complications.

RESULTS OF PRE-ECLAMPSIA

Pre-eclampsia is often associated with a disseminated intravascular coagulopathy, the placental thrombotic lesions occurring as a consequence of these coagulation disturbances often being microscopically and/or grossly visible. These placental infarcts appear to be associated with the presence of fibrin deposits in the interstitial spaces. In certain cases sufficient fibrin is accumulated to produce a true retroplacental haematoma. In addition, similar fibrin deposits are commonly found in other organs such as liver or brain. These findings encourage us to believe that the coagulation abnormalities observed are critical to the development of both maternal and foetal complications.

Placental microthrombotic lesions are, moreover, probably to a large part responsible for the changes in the blood flow velocities in maternal uterine arterial and foetal umbilical arterial circulations observed in IUGR, whether or not associated with maternal hypertension. Previously, research teams have attempted to treat pre-eclampsia with heparin; results have been either disappointing or at best transitory. In our opinion, this ineffectiveness may have been due to a relatively late initiation of therapy.

EFFECTS OF ASPIRIN AND DIPYRIDAMOLE

In one epidemiological study by Crandon (see Tables 1 and 2), it was reported that women who frequently used aspirin had a decreased incidence of gestational

Aspirin—towards 2000, edited by G. R. Fryers, 1990; Royal Society of Medicine Services International Congress and Symposium Series No. 168, published by Royal Society of Medicine Services Limited.

Table 1 *Characteristics of the trials with aspirin*

	A	B	C	D	E	F	G	H
Prospective	+	+	+	+	+	+	+	+
Randomization	+	+	−	+	+	+	+	+
Double-blind	−	+	−	+	+	+	+	+
Placebo control	−	+	−	+	+	+	+	+
End	84	86	86	88	89	?	?	89

A: (1)
B: (2)
C: (3)
D: (4)
E: Groupe Pergar. French Trial on persantine: leader Prof. C. Tchomoutsky, Paris
F: Groupe Epreda. French trial on aspirin and persantine: leader Prof. S. Uzan, Paris
G: CLASP. Collaborative Low-dose Aspirin Study in Pregnancy. (Dr M. de Swiet, Oxford)
H: USA. American trial at the National Institutes of Health, Bethesda. (Prof. B. Sibai)

hypertension or, if present, fewer additional complications such as pre-eclampsia. In fact, 11 years ago, we had decided to establish a study which examined the effectiveness of the combination of aspirin and dipyridamole in the prevention of pregnancy-induced hypertension complications. The majority of authors have utilized a small dosage of aspirin, <150 mg/day, in order to preserve the beneficial effects of prostacyclin. The second medication dipyridamole has been associated with aspirin in a number of studies. However, it has been difficult to distinguish its specific action from that of aspirin. Through its inhibition of phosphodiesterase it may potentiate the action of aspirin by retarding the destruction of adenosine monophosphate, thus making platelets more sensitive to prostacyclin. Dipyridamole may also have an autonomous action, stimulating a prostacyclin synthesis in platelets.

Table 2 *Criteria for inclusion, treatment regimen, onset, and number of patients for each trial*

	A	B	C	D	E	F	G	H
Criteria[a] for Inclusion	Nullipara Accid.[b] HTN[c]	IP Test with angio-tensin II	IUGR ⩾2	Doppler, But . . .	IUGR 1–2	IUGR 1–2	Past history	Primi gravida
Treatment 1								
Aspirin	150	150	60	150	0	150	60	65
Dipyridamole	300		225		225	225		
Treatment 2	0	P[d]	0	P	P	150	P	P
Treatment 3	—	—	—			P		—
Gestational age at onset of treatment	16	28	16	28–36	16	16	12–32	<24
No. patients	93	44	48	46	300	300	2000[e]	2000[e]
No. pregnancies	93	44	57	34+12	300	300		

[a]IUGR = intrauterine growth retardation
[b]'Accidental' previous pregnancy
[c]HTN = hypertension before pregnancy
[d]P = placebo
[e]Numbers expected, but . . .

We first conducted a review of the therapeutic trials using aspirin and/or dipyridamole (see Tables 1 and 2). It must be said that it is often difficult to separate out cases of IUGR that are secondary to vascular problems. For this reason, subsequent use of this term, IUGR, will include all foetuses without obvious malformation and in addition those of unknown aetiology. Twin pregnancies are excluded.

Concerning criteria for inclusion, study A has one principal fault, that of heterogeneous recruitment; a certain number of patients were even selected under the heading 'vascular risk'. Study B has an original and interesting selection process, in that it proposes a method for testing nulliparous women. Their criterion for inclusion is an increased sensitivity to angiotensin II challenge. Studies C, E and F use as the sole criterion for admission foetal weight related to gestational age at delivery. In our opinion this is the most logical selection process because the test is the only criterion which can be considered as objective. Moreover, the two French studies (E and F) include two types of patient, according to whether there have been one or two prior episodes of IUGR. This stratification attempts to identify future indications for therapy. Perhaps the benefits of therapy will be shown to outweigh the risks when the probability of recurrence is high, such as when there were two preceding pathological pregnancies.

The expression 'treatment used' means uniquely antiplatelet aggregation therapy; other more traditional antihypertensive medications are not specified.

The optimal dose: in our first study the treatment regimen of aspirin 150 mg/day with dipyridamole 300 mg/day was used, but it appeared that even smaller doses might be as effective.

Participation in studies such as these posed numerous ethical questions which were discussed at length by our ethics committee. The principal point of debate was whether it was appropriate to propose to women with a history of two prior pathological pregnancies that they start the third pregnancy with a possible placebo group. Others chose not to enter their patients into an internal control group because of their implicit belief in the following two arguments: that the efficacy of treatment was beyond any doubt (for our part this position was not sufficiently admissible); or that the treatment was innocuous, and this argument for us is also uncertain.

RESULTS OF EARLIER STUDIES

Comparing the results of the three trials (one by Beaufils and Uzan and two by Wallenburg) and focusing on the problem of IUGR, we see that there is a statistical difference for all the three studies. There is a reduction in the rate of IUGR and also a reduction in the rate of secondary complications. In our study there was a significant difference for *abruptio placentae,* which we consider a good indication for aspirin treatment.

In our study the duration of pregnancy at the time of delivery in the treatment group was increased significantly, whereas in the Wallenburg study it was 1–2 weeks shorter than the controls. This latter difference was not significant and, according to the author, the disparity between the two studies may in fact be explained by population differences with an unusually high incidence of prior uterine scar and repeated caesarean section in this treatment group when compared with the controls.

Placental examination in our study revealed reduced numbers of placental lesions and we demonstrated an improvement in plasma volume, plasma uric acid and platelet count. In all three studies, no haemorrhagic complications were noted in either mother or neonate, and no foetal malformations were observed in any of the treatment groups that could be attributed to the medication. In our study several patients receiving dipyridamole complained of headache, but these regressed rapidly with reduction of the dipyridamole dose; cessation of treatment was never required. However, it seems premature to conclude that the treatment regimen is innocuous. When considering the potential adverse effects of aspirin it is important to note that these medications do not generally modify the classical coagulation parameters except for those of platelet aggregation. In practice we used bleeding time, which is necessary to evaluate haemostatic changes in patients receiving low-dose aspirin. Significant prolongation of the bleeding time may occasionally be observed and in three cases we had bleeding time of >20 min with only 50 mg/day of aspirin. Moreover, after stopping aspirin therapy, a delay of 6–8 days was usually required for normalization of platelet function.

CONCLUSIONS

It is our belief that aspirin, and perhaps dipyridamole, will be shown to be an effective therapy in the prevention of IUGR in women who have had a prior, similarly complicated pregnancy and perhaps even more significantly effective in women with a history of two abnormal pregnancies. This treatment modality appears to be both effective and equally devoid of major risk, but controlled, randomized, double-blind studies with a placebo group are felt to be necessary before encouraging utilization of these medications.

This trial is now finished for inclusions in France and the last delivery will occur at the beginning of September, so that all our results should be ready by mid-November 1989.

REFERENCES

(1) Beaufils M, Uzan S. Prevention of pre-eclampsia by early platelet therapy. *Lancet* 1985; **i**: 840–2.
(2) Wallenburg HCS, Makovitz JW. Low-dose aspirin prevents pregnancy-induced hypertension and pre-eclampsia in angiotensin-sensitive primigravidae. *Lancet* 1986; **i**: 1–3.
(3) Wallenburg HC, Rotmans N. Prevention of recurrent idiopathic fetal growth retardation by low-dose aspirin and dipyridamole. *Am J Obstet Gynecol* 1987; **157**: 1230–5.
(4) Trudinger B, Cook CM, Thompson R, Giles W, Connelly A. Low-dose aspirin improves fetal weight in umbilical placental insufficiency. (Letter) *Lancet* 1988; **ii**: 214–5.

Aspirin in the prevention of stroke

Peter Sandercock

Department of Clinical Neurosciences, Western General Hospital, Edinburgh, UK

ANTIPLATELET TRIALISTS COLLABORATION

Data for establishing the role of aspirin and other antiplatelet agents in the prevention of stroke have been drawn from a meta-analysis prepared by the Antiplatelet Trialists Collaboration (APT). This international group of over 100 trialists consists of the principal investigators of randomized trials of antiplatelet agents in patients with different vascular diseases. It is a remarkable international group: there is complete data sharing, data are sent to the statistical secretariat in Oxford where they are audited and analysed centrally. All publications are in the name of the group as a whole. The clinical secretariat is based in Edinburgh and its main function is to serve as a register of all trials, both past and present, and it is extremely important to know about all the available data and not merely the published or selected data.

META-ANALYSIS OF CARDIOVASCULAR DISEASE STUDIES

By late 1986 there had been 25 randomized, controlled trials of antiplatelet agents in patients with transient ischaemic attack (TIA) or minor ischaemic stroke. Trials of antiplatelet agents had also taken place in patients with cardiac disease, that is survivors of myocardial infarction (MI), and patients with unstable angina. Patients with acute MI were not included in the analysis, so the results of ISIS II were excluded. The trials were all long-term, secondary prevention studies.

The conclusion from this analysis (published in the *British Medical Journal* in 1988) was that, in patients with cerebral and with cardiac disease, antiplatelet agents reduce the risk of stroke, MI or vascular death by about 25% (1). Many of the trials were individually unable to demonstrate this effect because they were too small, but certainly by looking at the totality of the evidence there was clear evidence of benefit.

That, however, was only a selection of the data that are available to us. There are in fact many more trials that have yet to be analysed. The prospective trial registry held in Edinburgh suggests that there are at least 130 randomized trials which have included a total of 126 000 patients or more. The trials have included patients with a wide variety of conditions: patients with unstable angina, coronary artery bypass grafting, atrial fibrillation, asymptomatic carotid bruit, peripheral

Aspirin—towards 2000, edited by G. R. Fryers, 1990; Royal Society of Medicine Services International Congress and Symposium Series No. 168, published by Royal Society of Medicine Services Limited.

vascular disease and diabetes. These are all patients who are at risk of stroke, so it would be of very considerable interest to know whether, in these trials as well, there is clear evidence of benefit from antiplatelet agents. The APT group is now obtaining these data.

There are several questions we hope to answer:

Is there a difference in treatment efficacy between males and females?

Does tolerance develop to the effect of aspirin or other antiplatelet agents? That is, is treatment as effective in the second and third years of treatment as it is in the first?

Is there a particular group in whom antiplatelet drugs are particularly effective in avoiding stroke, for example atrial fibrillation or peripheral vascular disease, or are antiplatelet agents equally effective in patients presenting with any kind of vascular disease?

Does the risk factor milieu of the patient influence the response to antiplatelet therapy?

Very importantly, particularly in the era of medical litigation, does aspirin cause cerebral haemorrhage which may be fatal or disabling?

Are the newer antiplatelet agents, such as ticlopidine, significantly more effective than aspirin or other antiplatelet agents?

What is the appropriate dose of aspirin for long-term secondary prevention?

Firstly, to deal with heterogeneity of treatment effect: That is, are antiplatelet drugs more effective in transient ischaemic attack (TIA) patients than in patients who have had a heart attack? One can say that there is no clear evidence of a difference yet, but that opinion is based only on two groups of patients; cerebrovascular disease and cardiac disease. It will obviously be of interest when the APT extends its analyses to look at other conditions, but at the moment the prevention of stroke with antiplatelet drugs appears approximately equal in patients presenting with cerebral or with cardiac disease.

Atrial fibrillation is an area of considerable research interest at the moment, stimulated by the recent publication of the Danish trial by Petersen *et al.* (2). This included 1000 patients with non-rheumatic atrial fibrillation who were randomly allocated between anticoagulants, aspirin 75 mg or matching placebo. The trial was unfortunately reported as negative with respect to aspirin, but this is not really the case because there is a high chance of a Type II error. That is, there was a reduction of about 20% in the risk of important vascular events in the aspirin group but, because of very small numbers of events there was a very considerable amount of uncertainty. This result is entirely compatible with the notion that, in patients with atrial fibrillation, aspirin might reduce the risk of important vascular events and emboli but there is uncertainty.

However, that trial is not the only one. There are now eight trials in progress on atrial fibrillation, some of which include a comparison between anticoagulants and antiplatelet drugs, while others include a comparison only with anticoagulants. A trial in Thailand, (Sitti-Amorn, personal communication) little known but very well executed, is comparing aspirin with placebo in patients with rheumatic heart disease but results are not yet available. There are also three trials being conducted comparing anticoagulants with placebo in atrial fibrillation and four trials which are comparisons between anticoagulants, aspirin and placebo. All of these trials are in progress and it will be of considerable interest when they are published to see whether aspirin will have a role in the prevention of stroke among patients with atrial fibrillation.

An issue of considerable concern at present is primary prevention of stroke. There have been two recent studies, one of which included 5000 British doctors (3) and the other 22 000 American doctors (4), comparing aspirin with no aspirin. The effect of aspirin on non-fatal MI in these studies is well known and is approximately the same as was seen in the secondary prevention trials reviewed in the APT meta-analysis. That is, all trials were compatible with approximately a 30% reduction in the risk of non-fatal MI. With respect to stroke, the position is rather different, and rather different indeed from the position in secondary prevention trials. In both trials, and in an overview of both primary prevention trials, there was a small but non-significant excess of strokes in patients treated with aspirin, which contrasts with the significant reduction observed in secondary prevention trials.

Why should this be? Stroke is not a homogeneous entity: it can be due to primary intracerebral haemorrhage; to cerebral infarction; to small vessel disease; to large vessel disease; or you may see infarction in the whole territory of the middle cerebral artery. Thus, one would not necessarily expect aspirin to be able equally to prevent all types of stroke, and it is even possible that aspirin might increase the risk of haemorrhagic stroke.

A meta-analysis of the published data suggests that aspirin, certainly in primary prevention, might increase the risk of haemorrhagic stroke approximately twofold, and the UK TIA aspirin study (5) again suggested that aspirin might increase the risk of cerebral haemorrhage. However, the numbers of events are extremely small and the confidence intervals thus extremely wide. We need to review the data collated by the APT to see whether this excess is real or not.

In the prevention of stroke and important vascular events a comparison of antiplatelet agents suggests that there is no important difference between antiplatelet regimens and that there is no important difference between higher and lower doses of aspirin. The choice of antiplatelet agent, therefore, in the prevention of stroke and heart attack, is more to do with side-effects and cost than with efficacy.

CONCLUSIONS

One should always remember that antiplatelet agents are part of the whole treatment of the patient. One has to remember that reduction of blood pressure is important, and that in a patient who has had a TIA or a stroke, reduction of diastolic blood pressure by 6 mmHg for a few years will reduce the risk of stroke by 43%. Cholesterol reduction will also reduce the risk of coronary heart disease events, as will antiplatelet therapy.

Antiplatelet therapy can prevent stroke in patients who have had some sort of vascular event, but whether aspirin should be used prophylactically against a first MI or stroke in patients who have not suffered any cardiovascular event is still uncertain, as are the effects of aspirin on cerebral haemorrhage.

REFERENCES

(1) Antiplatelet Trialists Collaboration. Secondary prevention of vascular disease by prolonged antiplatelet treatment. *Br Med J* 1988; **296**: 320–31.
(2) Petersen P, Boysen G, Gotfredson J, Andersen E, Andersen B. Placebo-controlled randomized trial of warfarin and aspirin for prevention of thromboembolic complications in chronic atrial fibrillation. *Lancet* 1989; **i**: 175–80.
(3) Peto R, Gray R, Collins R, *et al.* Randomized trial of prophylactic daily aspirin in British male doctors. *Br Med J* 1988; **296**: 313–16.
(4) Steering Committee of the Physicians' Health Study. Final Report of the aspirin component of the ongoing Physicians' Health Study. *N Engl J Med* 1989; **321**: 129–35.
(5) UK-TIA Study Group. United Kingdom transient ischaemic attack (UK-TIA) aspirin trial: interim results. *Br Med J* 1988; **296**:316–20.

DISCUSSION

Dr Lockhart: The recent Danish study by Petersen *et al.* used anticoagulation in post-myocardial infarction patients, and also investigated the effects on cerebrovascular accidents (1). They found a reduction of about 40% in cerebrovascular events with the use of warfarin. There were three deaths in the active therapy group compared with 16 deaths in the placebo group, but the three deaths happened to be haemorrhagic stroke. It may be that, although the incidence of these haemorrhagic events is very small, the incidence may be higher, but it appeared that using any kind of anticoagulation or antiplatelet therapy was still protective, because it seems that more strokes are ischaemic than haemorrhagic.

Dr Sandercock: The point is that it depends on the balance of risks and benefits. In secondary prevention there is clear evidence of net benefit in terms of stroke prevention. The difficulty is in primary prevention where the risks of having a stroke or a heart attack are much lower and therefore the balance of risks and benefits from having antiplatelet therapy may be rather different. There is uncertainty at the moment.

Professor de Gaetano: Dr Chalmers *et al.* have recently published another meta-analysis of studies with antiplatelet drugs in the prevention of stroke (2) and the results are different from those of the Antiplatelet Trialists Collaboration. Can you comment about the differences and why it should be so.

Dr Sandercock: It represents two different philosophies. Chalmers' approach is that you should only look at selected trials. Peto and I take the view that you should look at all truly randomized trials, whether published or unpublished. There is clear evidence from the Cancer Registry data by Simes published in the *Journal of Clinical Oncology* (3) showing that if you do a meta-analysis of only published trials, the results may be over-optimistic, and that if you examine both published and unpublished trials you will get a much more realistic assessment of treatment efficacy. If you want to apply the results of a meta-analysis, then you must have all trials, both published and unpublished.

The second point is that Chalmers excluded many of the trials that we used for reasons that are not clear. I believe we have more complete data than he does, and I believe that we have identified trials that he does not know about. For example, he did not include the Micristin study by Vogel *et al.* (4), which was done in the German Democratic Republic and published only in the conference proceedings. This study actually shows a far larger effect of aspirin than any other published study, but he did not identify that trial. I think it is extremely important that any meta-analysis should be based on all studies, published and unpublished, and I think his meta-analysis is open to many criticisms.

Professor Vermylen: I will be interested in your final data on peripheral vascular disease. Patients with intermittent claudication have very little risk of losing their limbs but they have a very high risk of dying from either myocardial infarction or stroke. At this point do you think it would be sensible to recommend aspirin prophylaxis in this group of patients?

Dr Sandercock: At the moment we do not have the overview data available for peripheral vascular disease. There have been a lot of trials in both peripheral vascular disease and lower limb vascular surgery, and it is all *sub judice* until we have analysed the results. It is very interesting that Collins has done a meta-analysis in deep venous thrombosis (Collins, personal communication) showing clear reductions in both pulmonary embolism and vascular death among patients at risk of deep venous thrombosis treated with aspirin as compared with placebo. I think we can draw from that the inference that in peripheral vascular disease it may well be that the same will hold true. But until we have actually examined the data and audited it, I am unable to speculate. One must think of the prevention of stroke, not just in transient ischaemic attack (TIA) patients but in all patients with vascular disease.

Professor Vermylen: Which dose of aspirin would you recommend at the present stage?

Dr Sandercock: Again, that is *sub judice*. The lowest dose that has been tested in the prevention of stroke, in a long-term secondary prevention trial, was the 300 mg used in the United Kingdom TIA aspirin study (referred to earlier). Lower doses are being tested; the Dutch trial (not yet published) is comparing 300 mg with 30 mg in patients with TIA and the results will be available in a year or two. The Swedish low-dose aspirin trial (not yet published) is testing lower doses and there are also low-dose trials in unstable angina. At the moment the lowest dose which is of proven efficacy in long-term secondary prevention is 300 mg, but further data will be available over the next two years on lower doses. At the moment I would say 300 mg but wait for further trials at lower doses.

Professor Vermylen: Do you think that the ISIS II study with 160 mg, although not a long-term study, gives very suggestive evidence that 160 mg would suffice?

Dr Sandercock: My philosophy would be that if a patient can tolerate 300 mg aspirin without side-effects, then they should be given that dosage. If they develop gastrointestinal side-effects which are, of course, dose-related, then the dose should be reduced, and 160 mg would be the next option. But I would always begin with 300 mg.

REFERENCES

(1) Petersen P, Boysen G, Gotfredson J, Andersen E, Andersen B. Placebo-controlled randomized trial of warfarin and aspirin for prevention of thromboembolic complications in chronic atrial fibrillation. *Lancet* 1989; **i**: 175–80.

(2) Sze P, Reitman D, Pinais M, Sacks HS, Chalmers TC. Antiplatelet agents in the secondary prevention of stroke: meta-analysis of the randomized control trials. *Stroke* 1988; **19**: 436–42.
(3) Simes R. Publication bias. The case for an international registry of clinical trials. *J Clin Oncol* 1986; **4**: 1529–41.
(4) Vogel G. Prevention of reinfarction with acetylsalicylic acid. In: Breddin K, *et al.* eds. *Prophylaxis of venous, peripheral, cardiac and cerebral events with acetylsalicylic acid*. Stuttgart: Schattaner Verlag, 1981: 123–8.

Aspirin and prevention of ischaemic artery disease

Chiara Cerletti and Giovanni de Gaetano

Consorzio Mario Negri Sud, Santa Maria Imbaro, Italy

EARLY STUDIES

We should not forget that possibly the first clinical trial on aspirin was published 33 years ago by a general practitioner working in California, in the *Mississippi Valley Medical Journal* (1). Dr Craven persuaded about 8000 of his patients and friends to take two tablets of aspirin a day as an antithrombotic agent and after 10 years of follow-up he wrote that not a single case of detectable coronary or cerebral thrombosis occurred among patients who had faithfully adhered to this regimen. It is interesting to realize that, at that time, neither Dr Craven, nor anyone else, knew anything about the effect of aspirin on platelets and cyclo-oxygenase or prostanoids. The basis on which Dr Craven's clinical trial was established was a vague similarity between the oral anticoagulant warfarin and aspirin and salicylate. He hoped to give his patients a less dangerous anticoagulant, in terms of haemorrhagic complications.

We know that aspirin has many other effects on haemostasis and on platelets, but we should not forget the many times in our experience that we utilize a false hypothesis for good experiments. Perhaps the hypothesis of cyclo-oxygenase and prostacyclin-thromboxane balance will also end up being a false hypothesis, but one which led to a number of interesting experiments providing interesting data.

We must analyse and judge the clinical efficacy of drugs; not in the way Dr Craven did, and perhaps even not in the way attributed to Galen. He wrote that: 'All who drink of this remedy recover in a short time except those whom it does not help, who all die. Therefore, it is obvious that it fails only in incurable cases.'

META-ANALYSIS

The meta-analysis is a very important means of understanding the mechanisms and measuring the degree of clinical efficacy of drugs. Considering all vascular events in the Antiplatelet Trialists Collaboration (ATC) meta-analysis (2), a significant reduction of 20–22% in vascular events was observed, and this was true even if the qualifying event was cerebrovascular, a myocardial infarction or unstable angina. Out of the 25 trials involved in the analysis at least 19 used

Aspirin—towards 2000, edited by G. R. Fryers, 1990; Royal Society of Medicine Services International Congress and Symposium Series No. 168, published by Royal Society of Medicine Services Limited.

aspirin, so the data derived from the ATC can be safely applied to aspirin, and not only to antiplatelet treatment in general.

RISKS AND BENEFITS

If one only considers vascular mortality, one finds a less evident but still significant effect. It is very important that non-vascular deaths were not modified by antiplatelet treatment. This suggests that aspirin, or any other antiplatelet treatments utilized in these trials, did not affect the vascular mortality in a non-specific way. There is always the danger that a panacea can give a wrong result, because you only consider one aspect of the programme. In fact there was no effect at all on non-vascular mortality. Interestingly, if one translates the percentage reduction to actual figures, they show that a 25% reduction means that, among 100 patients treated for two years with aspirin or another antiplatelet agent, one fatal and two non-fatal events will be avoided.

This is a very important result, because if these data are extrapolated to all the potential individuals who can benefit from this treatment, the numbers become very important. However, we should consider that 97 out of these 100 patients will receive treatment without any apparent benefit, because about 90 of them will not die, independent of any treatment they will receive, and seven will die despite the fact that they have taken aspirin for two years. So although we are especially interested in the three patients who received the benefit from aspirin, in future we should pay much more attention to the non-responders in these trials. We collect thousands of patients, but we are only interested in patients who respond positively to any given treatment. I think we shall learn much more about the mechanism of action of drugs, the real efficacy of the treatment, if we consider the problem of non-responders.

Unfortunately, at the present moment we are unable to identify the three patients who will benefit from aspirin, so we are obliged to give the drug to 100 patients, knowing that only three of them will receive an advantage. Since every active treatment may produce adverse effects, we must consider very carefully the value of giving a treatment which will provide no benefit but which can produce some untoward effects. Thus, the problem of excessive enthusiasm about antiplatelet treatment should be critically considered, and much effort should be paid to understanding which patients will benefit, from a clinical point of view, through a treatment which, from a biochemical point of view, is similar in everybody.

ASPIRIN DOSAGE

When the meta-analysis by the ATC is considered in terms of the different drugs, no significant difference is seen between the different doses of aspirin utilized. Even 1.5 g aspirin/day or 300 mg/day gave results which could not be statistically distinguished. It is a serious problem if we consider the hypothesis of prostacyclin and thromboxane balance and relate this to the concept of low dose aspirin selectively affecting platelet function.

In about 60 of the patients in the UK Transient Ischaemic Attack (UK-TIA) study (3) we measured a number of coagulation, platelet and prostanoid parameters. The study had one placebo group, one group with relatively low-dose aspirin (300 mg/day) and a group with high-dose aspirin (1.2 g/day). Platelet aggregation was similarly prevented by the two aspirin treatments; there was complete suppression of arachidonate-induced platelet aggregation by both regimens. The only difference we could find between the two groups of patients treated with different doses of aspirin were the levels of salicylate. Patients in the high-dose group had about 3–4 times more salicylate at a steady state level in the blood as compared with the low-dose aspirin group. In contrast, bleeding time and suppression of serum thromboxane were similarly affected. Interestingly, in spite of the fact that these patients took aspirin 1.2 g/day for months or years, there was no modification of the urinary excretion of 6-keto-$PGF_{1\alpha}$ or thromboxane.

These clinical data should raise some doubts about the clinical relevance of the prostacyclin/thromboxane balance: why, if patients have taken so much aspirin every day, should they excrete the same amount of 6-keto-$PGF_{1\alpha}$, the metabolite of prostacyclin, compared to low-dose aspirin or to placebo?

Aspirin has been considered a drug that, when given to man or animal, produces a scientific paper. However, it also produces salicylate and the hypothesis has been advanced that in fact peripheral vessels and peripheral organs mainly come into contact with salicylate, not aspirin, because of the de-acetylation during gastrointestinal absorption and first pass hepatic de-acetylation (4). In experimental animals, we showed that aspirin comes into contact with platelets and with pre-systemic vessels, but peripheral vessels and renal tissues mainly come into contact with salicylate (5). This is the main reason why, despite ingestion of high doses of aspirin, it is very difficult to demonstrate any reduction in the urinary products of prostaglandins produced within the kidney. Measuring the urinary excretion of prostanoids may not therefore be a good marker for what happens in the circulation and in the pre-systemic vessels when aspirin is ingested.

Data from Carlo Patrono's group (6) show how complicated may be the effect of a single dose of aspirin, even a very low dose. If one considers four parameters in the same group of individuals, there is complete suppression of platelet thromboxane, and no effect at all on urinary 6-keto-$PGF_{1\alpha}$ excretion. However, measuring the metabolites of either thromboxane or prostacyclin which derive from a mixed source of systemic and pre-systemic vessels, one sees an intermediate biochemical effect. Thus, it is quite difficult to answer the question: what does aspirin do on vascular walls at a given dose or in a given formulation? It depends on where you measure the metabolites and which kind of metabolites you detect. The effect of the same dose of aspirin in the same patient may appear completely different and this should be taken into account when we discuss the clinical efficacy of aspirin. We do not yet understand very clearly why the clinical data do not correspond exactly with our experimental or clinical pharmacological results.

Another interesting study we performed with Dr Prentice in Leeds (7) showed that three parameters, fibrinogen levels, fibrinopeptide-A which is a marker of activation of coagulation of the haemostatic system, and haemoglobin, were significantly reduced in a group of patients taking a high dose of aspirin. We know that reducing fibrinogen can be a good way to reduce cerebrovascular or cardiovascular disease. A reduction of haematocrit is also an important means of reducing the thrombogenicity of platelets and the thrombogenicity of the haemostatic system. Reduction of fibrinopeptide-A could also be a marker of inhibition of the coagulation system.

We should not forget that early report by Dr Craven which suggested that aspirin may act *also* as an anticoagulant: perhaps at very high doses such as those used in that particular group of patients a small anticoagulant effect related, not to the acetyl group, but to the anticoagulant property of salicylate, could play a minimal but perhaps interesting role.

Therefore, I would propose this as a provocative hypothesis: the fact that in the UK-TIA trial there was no difference between the two doses of aspirin could be due in part to the fact that high-dose aspirin might have had a beneficial effect because of mechanisms unrelated to inhibition of platelet cyclo-oxygenase activity. We should ask whether reduction of haemoglobin, fibrinogen and fibrinopeptide-A could then be considered a side-effect of aspirin, or a therapeutic mode of action of aspirin, at least at high doses.

THE UNITY OF ATHEROSCLEROTIC DISEASE

Non-fatal stroke in the ATC meta-analysis (2) was reduced significantly, not only in patients with a previous cerebrovascular accident but even more in patients with myocardial infarction (MI), so secondary prevention of MI can be associated with a primary prevention of stroke in patients with MI. This is a very interesting basic hypothesis, which suggests that patients seen by cardiologists, neurologists or other specialists are clinical artefacts, that we should perhaps consider the patients affected by vascular disease as a whole, not distinguishing whether the first clinical manifestation of a basic atherosclerotic disease is at a cardiac, cerebral or even peripheral level.

This is an interesting hypothesis which is currently being tested in Italy by the PLAT group (Progetto Lombardo Atero Trombosi) (18). We have collected about 1000 patients with cerebral, cardiac or peripheral disease as a qualifying event and we are trying to determine whether we can consider these patients as a unique group who can benefit from the same therapy, or if the patient with a primary manifestation at cardiac level is substantially different from a patient whose first clinical manifestation is at cerebral or peripheral level.

It is interesting that in the ISIS II trial (9), patients given aspirin (160 mg daily) starting very early after acute MI enjoyed very similar results to those of the ATC meta-analysis (2) (the latter did not receive aspirin until two months after the event). Also, patients from the ISIS II trial treated with aspirin enjoyed a significant, very important reduction not only in non-fatal reinfarction, which was reduced by 31%, but also in non-fatal stroke which was reduced by 42% in the meta-analysis of 10 trials of long-term treatment, and by about 45% in the ISIS II trial. Perhaps the manifestation of prevention of a cerebral accident follows the same pathogenetic mechanism in patients with a previous MI history or with a very recent MI, and one should also ask the question whether, based on the particular method of selecting patients in the ISIS II trial, a number of patients with unstable angina, not MI, were involved, and whether this beneficial effect on cerebrovascular accident (CVA) also applies to angina patients. This was not the case in the two earlier trials of angina patients; there was no reduction of CVA, so we have here clinical data which still need to be considered altogether and to be analysed more critically, in order to suggest hypotheses and new interpretations, both from a therapeutic and a physiological point of view.

AMERICAN PHYSICIANS' TRIAL

Consider also the American Physicians' trial (10) where, if platelets play the same pathogenetic part in MI and in cerebral stroke, one should have expected at least similar results in preventing MI and stroke. In fact this was not the case because MI was significantly reduced by aspirin, while stroke, either fatal or non-fatal, was not affected. The question arises whether the role of platelets in myocardial infarction and stroke is different in patients with clinically manifest atherosclerosis, or whether there is no role in patients without atherosclerosis, or without clinical manifestations. If platelets have no role, why should aspirin prevent MI in apparently healthy people? Is aspirin perhaps working in this trial in a different way from that seen in trials on patients with already manifest disease? This is an open question to which there is not yet an answer. Certainly there is enough incentive for further investigation.

When we analyse in more detail the mortality data in the American Physicians trial we also find another disturbing result. The patients classified under sudden death were more numerous in the aspirin group than in the control group. Here the figures are very low so we cannot extend discussion too far. However, one should consider that sudden death did not show the same clinical benefit that was found with MI. This is disturbing in view of the data which generated a lot of enthusiasm among many people published a few years ago by Davies and Thomas (11), in 100 patients who died of sudden death. In 95 of these 100 patients a thrombus, mainly a platelet thrombus, was found at autopsy. Thus the idea that sudden death was mainly an electrical kind of death was challenged and many people believed that sudden death could be a clinical end of a platelet-based thrombus. If that is so, why does aspirin prevent mortality due to MI, and not fatality due to sudden death? Either we have to revise and rediscuss these anatomical pathological data, which are very impressive, or we have to try and understand why MI and sudden death behave clinically in such a different way.

We should not forget that the subjects who participated in the American Physicians' trial were very healthy people, and this generates some doubt about the relevance of these data to a general population. However, it gives us important information; it tells us that even if we eliminate all the risk factors, as was done in this selection of population, if we select very healthy people, with low serum cholesterol, no diabetes, no hypertension and so on, still aspirin and antiplatelet treatment can have some benefit. So the campaign we have to undertake to reduce risk factors is not in contradiction to a pharmacological approach with an antiplatelet drug.

CONCLUSIONS

I believe that more accurate selection of patients, especially those with cerebrovascular disease, could in future years demonstrate a greater therapeutic benefit of aspirin. Earlier initiation of therapy with aspirin after the ischaemic event could also help to select more responsive patients. I believe that any dose of aspirin <300 mg/day is good, on the basis of what we know at the moment. I suggest we undertake a trial of aspirin at any dose against other treatments and I believe that we need more significant and more convincing data on primary prevention and on the combination of aspirin with other treatments. Finally, and I leave this question as something we should keep in the back of our minds, perhaps a mechanism of aspirin different from cyclo-oxygenase inhibition should also be taken into account (5,12).

REFERENCES

(1) Craven LL. Experience with aspirin (acetylsalicylic acid) in the non-specific prophylaxis of coronary thrombosis. *Mississippi Valley Med J* 1953; **75**: 38–44.

(2) Antiplatelet Trialists' Collaboration. Secondary prevention of vascular disease by prolonged antiplatelet treatment. *BMJ* 1988; **296**: 320–31.
(3) UK-TIA Study Group. United Kingdom transient ischemic attack (UK-TIA) aspirin trial: Interim results. *BMJ* 1988; **296**: 316–20.
(4) Hampton KK, Loizou LA, Cerletti C, *et al.* Coagulation, fibrinolytic and platelet function in patients on long term therapy with aspirin 300 mg or 1200 mg daily compared with placebo. *Thromb Haemost* 1990 (in press).
(5) de Gaetano G, Cerletti C, Dejana E, Latini R. Platelets and vascular occlusion. Pharmacology of platelet inhibition in humans: Implications of the salicylate-aspirin interaction. *Circulation* 1985; **72**: 1185–93.
(6) Cerletti C, Gambino MC, Garattini S, de Gaetano G. Biochemical selectivity of oral versus intravenous aspirin in rats. Inhibition by oral aspirin of cyclo-oxygenase activity in platelets and presystemic but not systemic vessels. *J Clin Invest* 1986; **78**: 323–6.
(7) Patrignani P. Aspirin as a selective inhibitor of platelet cyclo-oxygenase in man. *XXII Congress of the International Society of Hematology*, 1988. Abs. Sym F-4-2: 93.
(8) Roncaglioni MC, Reyers I, Cerletti C, Donati MB, de Gaetano G. Moderate anticoagulation by salicylate prevents thrombosis without bleeding complications. An experimental study in rats. *Biochem Pharmacol* 1988; **37**: 4743–5.
(9) ISIS-2 Collaborative Group. Randomised trial of intravenous streptokinase, oral aspirin, both or neither among 17 189 cases of suspected acute myocarddial infarction. *Lancet* 1988; **ii** 349–60.
(10) Steering Committee of the Physicians' Health Study Research Group. Final report on the aspirin component of the ongoing physician's health study. *N Engl J Med* 1989; **321**: 129–35.
(11) Davies MJ, Thomas AC. Thrombosis and acute coronary artery lesions in sudden cardiac ischaemic death. *N Engl J Med* 1984; **310**: 1137–40.
(12) Cerletti C, Carriero MR, de Gaetano G. Platelet aggregation response to single or paired aggregating stimuli after low-dose aspirin. *N Engl J Med* 1986; **314**: 316–8.

Aspirin and immunity: Modulation of lymphokine production

Allan L. Goldstein

Department of Biochemistry and Molecular Biology,
The George Washington University Medical Center, Washington DC, USA

INTRODUCTION

For the past 25 years I have been interested primarily in the cell-mediated wing of the immune system; the component of the immune system that is controlled by the thymus gland, which is the master gland of the immune system. We now know from the results of many studies that the thymus controls the maturation and differentiation of a variety of T-cells that provide us with much of our immunity to viruses, mycobacteria, fungi and tumours. We know also from recent studies that some of the peptides isolated from the thymus which have hormone-like properties, such as the thymosins, in addition to influencing the immune system, can also feed back, control and modulate hormones produced by the pituitary. This thymus-brain connection is one of the most interesting new areas of neuro-immunology.

About 10 years ago, during the course of studies that we were carrying out with the thymosins, attempting to learn more about their mechanism of action, we decided to look at the group of agents such as the cyclo-oxygenase inhibitors, as well as a number of other agents, to determine whether they might influence or inhibit the effects of the thymic peptides. That was how we got into the area that now is very much involved with aspirin and other cyclo-oxygenase inhibitors.

THE IMMUNE SYSTEM

The immune system is very complicated and, in addition to the thymus, it includes the bone marrow, a variety of cell populations of which there are various sub-sets of T-cells, the macrophage which plays an important role, and the B-cells. Furthermore, the system becomes much more complicated when we now know that the assignable mediators of the immune system include a large number of hormonal-like molecules called lymphokines and cytokines, ranging from interleukin-1 (IL-1) to interleukin II to the interferons, to the colony stimulating factors. There are dozens of molecules which, in essence, are the new medicines that are being studied with great potential in the clinic. It is interesting to me, therefore, that one of the oldest medicines, aspirin,

Aspirin—towards 2000, edited by G. R. Fryers, 1990; Royal Society of Medicine Services International Congress and Symposium Series No. 168, published by Royal Society of Medicine Services Limited.

appears to fit within the scheme of things and might actually play a role in this process.

THYMOSIN

My laboratory was involved in the first clinical trials in the USA with a calf thymic hormone preparation, thymosin, which consisted of a family of peptide molecules that have now been sequenced. Several have been synthesized and are currently in clinical trials. The first clinical studies took place at UCLA Medical Center in a girl who was born without a functioning thymus gland, as were several children with this particular life-threatening disease, a form of Digeorge syndrome. Since we first started using these peptides clinically in the mid-1970s, many of the biological response modifiers, as they are known, have already found an important place in clinical medicine and we will hear a lot more about others in the future. Our studies would suggest that aspirin might play an important role in combination with some of these biological response modifiers, and perhaps with other agents, to regulate the immune system more effectively.

From the calf thymus gland we were able to isolate, characterize, sequence and synthesize varieties of these immune peptides that we call thymosins, using recombinant and solid phase peptide synthesis techniques, and we are using them experimentally to study a number of indications associated with immune deficiencies. The thymosins can augment lymphokine production such as interferon-α, for example, and they can also augment the production of γ-interferon as well as a variety of other lymphokines.

ROLE OF THE EICOSANOIDS

The eicosanoids have a role in lymphocyte mitogenesis. It is clear that the lipoxygenases and cyclo-oxygenases, which are prostaglandin intermediates, play important roles in maturation and functioning of various T-cell populations as well as other immune populations. It was from the observations that prostaglandins played such an important part in lymphocyte function that we first began 10 years ago to look at the effects of agents like aspirin. We found that aspirin has a profound effect on lymphokine production. One of the first studies we undertook was to determine the effects *in vitro* on human lymphocytes of aspirin and salicylic acid, and study its effects on lymphokine production, using peripheral blood lymphocytes. We showed that aspirin *in vitro* could modulate or increase the production of a lymphokine such as γ-interferon, where salicylic acid was without effect. We originally introduced these agents to see if they could inhibit the functions of the thymosins on these same cells and we found that just the opposite occurred.

We believe that the T-cell produces many of the lymphokines such as IL-2 and these T-cells are extensively influenced by another cell population, the macrophages. The macrophage produces agents such as IL-1, which provides one of the first signals to the T-cell, but it also produces a lot of prostaglandins. From the results of several studies it is quite clear that the effect of aspirin at the level of up-regulation of these lymphokines is by inhibiting cyclo-oxygenase of the macrophage, and that the macrophage plays a key role in whether or not lymphokine production is suppressed. In other words, under normal circumstances prostaglandins can down-regulate T-cell immune responses.

This also suggests that other cells such as cancer cells, which produce significant quantities of prostaglandins, might spread and be deleterious to the host because, in the process of growing, they secrete prostaglandins. The end-effect of that is to down-regulate the very immune system with which the body tries to fight these cancer cells. We believe that this observation, which deals with normal regulation of the immune system, may have a place in other areas as well. If you deprive the peripheral blood lymphocytes of the macrophage, you lose the ability to make γ-interferon, the aspirin effect or the thymosin effect, which can only be restored if you return that macrophage to the cell population.

IN VIVO STUDIES

From other studies following our *in vitro* work we began to investigate the effects of oral aspirin 325 mg on peripheral blood lymphocytes, on the ability to produce certain lymphokines such as IL-2. Oral aspirin very quickly stimulates the production of IL-2 by PHA-stimulated lymphocytes, reaching a maximum within 10 h, and γ-interferon which reaches a peak at about 24 h in normal individuals. One of the side-effects of conventional therapy on a tumour mass, whether it is chemotherapy, radiotherapy or surgery, is suppression of host immunity. One of the greatest potentials of the biological response modifiers of the immune modulators is to restore some of that systemic host immunity, and many of the biological response modifiers that are being studied are being given now in combination with conventional therapies as a way to overcome some of the suppressive effects of immunity. It may very well be that some day aspirin will be considered in the same situation.

It is very clear to us that aspirin, as well as the thymosins, is an effective biological response modifier, and both appear to have additive effects on lymphokine production. It is also clear that the thymosins act by a different mechanism than does aspirin, so that there is a real potential for combination studies.

CLINICAL STUDIES

Two years ago we began to apply this new information about aspirin in a clinical setting. We asked the questions:

1. Are the immunomodulatory effects we are seeing anecdotally, sustainable in a randomized, placebo-controlled trial of aspirin?
2. Is it possible to use this information to intervene in a very common ailment, namely the common cold?

My colleagues at the George Washington University Medical Center and associates from the University of Virginia School of Medicine undertook to study this question in a group of young medical students. Clinically we found that we clearly could not cure the common cold. From this small study there was no impact on the cold following introduction of a virus nasally, but we did see under controlled circumstances very interesting changes with regard to the immune system in what was the first randomized trial of aspirin in this setting. There is no question that aspirin had a very positive effect in modulating immune responses. We used the rhinovirus, which is a non-envelope virus with single-stranded RNA, two receptor families and many sub-strains. Medical students were tested first to see whether they had ever met this sub-strain before and individuals with a titre greater than 1 : 2 were excluded. Nine subjects received aspirin 325 mg and nine received matching placebo on days 1, 3 and 5; virus on day 2; and they were then isolated. We studied a variety of immune parameters, viral titres and blastogenesis.

There was no difference between aspirin or placebo with regard to virus shedding, seroconversion or other symptoms. Unfortunately, but typically in this type of experimentally-induced virus, the normal 50–80% take was reached in the aspirin group but not in the placebo group. Looking at nasal mucus production there was no difference between the groups. However, some potentially very interesting findings are now guiding us in future studies.

1. It was very clear, and has been seen before with regard to infection, that by day 6 there was a significant increase in blood cortisol levels.
2. Also, for the first time under controlled conditions in acute infection, we found that the thymosin-α_1 levels as measured by radioimmunoassay were markedly elevated by day 6 and the effect could even be seen earlier.

By day 2 of the trial, under controlled circumstances, we saw a significant increase in γ-interferon and IL-2 production in the students receiving aspirin. In addition, over and above the maximum stimulation seen with regard to interferon and IL-2, when we added thymosin *in vitro* to the lymphocytes from these individuals, we saw an increase in lymphokine production. Thus, as we had seen previously in an uncontrolled study, there was an added effect of thymosin *in vitro*.

CONCLUSIONS

Our conclusions from this study are that:

1. Aspirin did not alter the incidence or clinical course of experimental rhinovirus colds using this protocol and this small but randomized, well-studied group.
2. Oral aspirin stimulates production of IL-2 and γ-interferon by peripheral blood leucocytes and, following oral aspirin, thymosin further stimulates production of both lymphokines *in vitro*.

The fact that under controlled circumstances we could clearly modulate lymphokine production in a positive way will, we believe, be important and should be pursued in different settings.

FUTURE RESEARCH

Some of the questions now being pursued include:

1. Does aspirin augment immune function in the elderly and in other immuno-suppressed populations?

There is no question that aspirin is an effective immune modulator, at least in regard to lymphokine production in a young healthy medical student, but what does it do in elderly populations whose immune systems are suppressed?

Can we, by modifying their immune responses, enable them to deal better with normal host resistance?

2. Can aspirin speed recovery from immunosuppressive treatment for cancer or inflammatory illnesses?

This is an area of keen interest because tumours produce a lot of prostaglandins and there is no question that, in general, high doses of prostaglandins are not good for the immune system.

3. Will aspirin have a future role as an adjuvant to conventional anti-tumour treatment?

These observations emerged from our initial quest, not to study aspirin *per se* but to try and find a way to study a thymic peptide in which we were interested. We believe we have come across a potential new indication for aspirin, and it is very important now for us to follow up these observations, both by further animal studies and by well-controlled clinical studies, to see if the modulation of lymphokine responses can be translated into a clinical setting that is characterized by an immune balance or an immune suppression.

DISCUSSION

Dr Pozzilli: We have found that gene expression *in vitro* may be induced by different factors in peripheral lymphocytes. You have shown, *in vitro* and *in vivo*, that aspirin may increase some cytokine production and I was particularly interested in the data showing an increase of cortisol that was also seen in placebo-controlled patients. If you suggest that aspirin may have an effect on lymphokine production, and thymosin fraction may even increase this effect, it is possible that this could be mediated directly through production of adrenocorticotrophic hormone (ACTH) by lymphocytes. We do not have to assume that cortisol is only stimulated by the pituitary; it could be stimulated direct by lymphocytes. I would like to know whether you have any data on the possible effect on release of cytokines, ACTH and other peptides, by lymphocytes.

Professor Goldstein: Only the lack of time prevented me from discussing the neuroendocrine component. One of the major discoveries in the field of immunology during the last few years has been the observation that lymphocytes themselves are capable of producing peptides which we thought at one time to be produced only by the pituitary, and these include not only β-endorphin, but ACTH, thyroid-stimulating hormone (TSH), growth hormone, a variety of very interesting molecules and these new connections between T-cells and the pituitary have really brought into focus the fact that we have a very integrated circuit between the two systems. It has been proposed by Blalock and Smith and others (1) that some of these neuroendocrine responses of the T-cells are related to the ability of the immune system to respond to agents that you cannot detect. The physiological significance of those, why the T-cells are making these molecules, still has to be established, but it is correct that they do. We have not looked at the effects of aspirin on the production of ACTH, β-endorphin, or any others of these molecules, but it would be a very worth-while experiment to undertake because it might help to explain some other effects of aspirin that have to do with actions that are thought currently to occur at the level of the central nervous system.

REFERENCE

Smith EM, Phar M, Kruger TE, Coppenhauer DH, Blalock JE. Human lymphocyte production of immunoreactive thyrotropin. *Proc Natl Acad Sci USA* 1983; **80**: 6010–3.

Immunosuppression in irradiated breast cancer patients: *In vitro* effect of cyclo-oxygenase inhibitors

Jerzy Wasserman[1] in collaboration with G. Wolk[1], B. Petrini[1], O. Strannegard[1], I. Vedin[1], H. Blomgren[2] and U Glas[3]

[1]Central Microbiological Laboratory of Stockholm County Council, Sweden,
[2]Radiumhemmet, Karolinska Institute and Hospital, Stockholm, Sweden,
[3]Department of Oncology Sodersjukhuset, Stockholm, Sweden

IMMUNE SYSTEM CHANGES

Local irradiation therapy is widely used as an adjuvant to surgery in the treatment of primary breast cancer. Prospective randomized trials have shown that this treatment prevents the development of local regional metastases. However, it does not seem to reduce the development of distant metastases or prolong survival of the patients. Since irradiation therapy may cause a profound lymphopenia, we considered it important to investigate in detail the changes of the immune system which occur after irradiation for breast cancer. In addition we wanted to examine if there is any relationship between the prognosis of the patients and the extent of the irradiation-induced immunosuppression.

Our studies confirmed that local irradiation therapy for breast cancer consisting of 45 Gy causes a severe lymphopenia with reductions of both T- and non-T-lymphocytes. The non-T-lymphocytes were depressed to the higher relative extent but their recovery was more rapid, within six months. Recovery of the T-cell population appeared to proceed much more slowly. Recent studies have shown that it is still incomplete 10–11 years after irradiation therapy. Our studies took place in three groups of patients: non-irradiated patients, patients who were irradiated preoperatively, and patients who were irradiated postoperatively. Even 10–11 years after irradiation, patients still have significantly fewer lymphocytes, T-lymphocytes and T-helper cells. T-suppressor cells were reconstituted by that time, or even earlier.

Several lymphocyte functions measured on a cell-for-cell basis were also found to be changed after irradiation. So was the mitogen-induced production of immunoglobulins *in vitro*, both of IgM and IgG, significantly reduced after irradiation. Also mitogenic responses of lymphocytes to polyclonal mitogens and specific antigens were depressed.

The impaired lymphoproliferative responses observed following irradiation were found to be due to non-specific suppressor cells with characteristics of monocytes.

Aspirin—towards 2000, edited by G. R. Fryers, 1990; Royal Society of Medicine Services International Congress and Symposium Series No. 168, published by Royal Society of Medicine Services Limited.

We could also demonstrate that irradiation therapy increased oxidative metabolism of the individual monocytes as measured by capacity to reduce nitroblue-tetrazolium. Since activated monocytes are known to produce a number of arachidonic acid metabolites of both the cyclo-oxygenase and lipoxygenase pathways, we tried to examine in more detail the role of monocytes in immuno-suppression after irradiation, and also to find out whether the suppression could be explained by the increased biosynthesis of prostaglandins. Some of these prostaglandins are very well known to be strongly immunosuppressive.

The reactivity to tuberculin after irradiation was significantly depressed. Adding indomethacin gave increased reactivity by approximately 0.25 $\log_{10}$ units. Adding silica had the same effect; the monocytes were inactivated. The results could be interpreted in two ways: either the biosynthesis of the immunosuppressive prostaglandins by monocytes is increased after irradiation therapy, or the sensitivity of the lymphocytes to prostaglandins is increased.

LYMPHOCYTE SENSITIVITY

We compared the sensitivity of lymphocytes to prostaglandins D_2 and E_2 in breast cancer patients and normal controls; there was no difference. We then looked for the sensitivity of lymphocytes to prostaglandins E_2 and D_2 at the completion of therapy, and three and six months after the completion of therapy. There was no increased sensitivity to prostaglandins. Thus, the conclusions drawn from these studies were that local irradiation therapy for breast cancer not only causes long-standing lymphopenia but also activates monocytes to increase biosynthesis of prostaglandins which suppress immunological responses of T-cells.

EFFECTS OF CYCLO-OXYGENASE INHIBITORS

Subsequently, a number of experiments were performed to examine more systematically the effects of various cyclo-oxygenase inhibitors on mitogenic responses of non-purified lymphocyte preparations to different concentrations of phytohaemagglutinin (PHA). Although the results varied substantially between different tests, our general conclusion was that all the inhibitors tested—indomethacin, meclofenamic acid and lysine-mono-acetylsalicylate (Aspisol)—may to a varying extent increase mitogenic responses of lymphocytes from control individuals when present in the culture at concentrations ranging from 10^{-7}–10^{-5} molar.

In order to examine the role of monocytes, experiments were performed in which non-purified and purified lymphocytes from the same donors were stimulated with PHA in the presence of various inhibitors. When purified lymphocytes were used, the cyclo-oxygenase inhibitors indomethacin, meclofenamic acid and acetylsalicylic acid had very little effect as far as their reactivity to PHA was concerned. On the other hand, when using non-purified lymphocytes, which means lymphocyte preparations containing mono-cytes, cyclo-oxygenase inhibitors had a rather pronounced effect in terms of increased reactivity; this was so for both indomethacin and meclofenamic acid with a lesser effect as far as acetylsalicylic acid is concerned. This observation suggested that monocytes and not lymphocytes were the main producers of immunosuppressive metabolites of arachidonic acid. However, we cannot exclude a role for thrombocytes in this context, as the cell preparations were contaminated to some degree by thrombocytes.

RELATIONSHIP BETWEEN PROGNOSIS AND IMMUNOLOGICAL REACTIVITY AFTER RADIATION THERAPY

We were interested in the relationship between prognosis and immunological reactivity after irradiation therapy. During the years 1971–1974, we examined the PHA and the purified protein derivative (PPD) responses of blood lymphocytes from 114 breast cancer patients who received local irradiation therapy, 45 Gy, as adjuvant to surgery. They were included in a prospective randomized trial taking place at the Karolinska Hospital, Stockholm, aiming at determining the clinical value of pre- and postoperative irradiation. Mitogen responses of blood lymphocytes were determined before radiation therapy and at various time intervals after its completion. After a clinical follow-up period of 10–13 years, we analysed the results to determine whether there was any relationship between mitogen responses and survival of patients. There was no detectable association between the initial PHA and PPD reactivity and survival of the patient but, on the other hand, mortality was significantly higher among patients with low post-irradiation PHA and PPD reactivity.

Patients were divided into two groups: good responders who had a PPD and PHA activity higher than the median value, and those who were poor responders, with a reactivity lower than the median value. The mortality was significantly higher for poor PPD and PHA reactors. This applies to PPD reactivity at the completion of irradiation, PHA reactivity at the completion of irradiation, and to PPD reactivity 6–10 months after irradiation. This trend existed irrespective of the lymph node status in the axilla.

In order to elucidate further the relation of PPD and PHA reactivity to prognosis, regardless of the clinical stage, a log rank analysis of survival was performed in which both patient groups were stratified for the stage. This analysis demonstrated a higher survival for patients with high PPD reactivity during the first eight years of the observation period, also after the clinical stage had been considered.

We drew the following conclusion from these studies. Adjuvant local irradiation therapy for breast cancer is of clinical value, since it reduces development of original occurrences. However, it does not seem to improve patient survival significantly. This may be due to the fact that the treatment sharply reduces the size, and several functions, of the lymphocyte pool of the body. It means that the natural immune defence against residual cancer cells may be weakened. It is possible that the beneficial effects of irradiation treatment may be overshadowed by the detrimental effect on the immune system. We believe that it would be worth while to investigate whether the clinical value of the treatment can be improved if the irradiation-induced suppression of lymphocyte responses is reduced to a minimum.

Since this can be proved *in vitro* with cyclo-oxygenase inhibitors it is possible that this can also be achieved *in vivo* with such drugs. Several drugs such as meclofenamic acid, acetylsalicyclic acid, lysine-mono-acetylsalicylate, indomethacin and diclofenac sodium inhibit prostaglandin synthesis. In order to choose the most suitable drug which could be used in an eventual study we compared various cyclo-oxygenase inhibitors with respect to their capacity to reverse irradiation-induced suppression of mitogen response.

Twenty consecutive female patients with breast cancer treated postoperatively with local irradiation therapy served as lymphocyte donors. Lymphocytes dropped sharply at completion of irradiation, but monocytes did not. The reactivity to PHA of lymphocytes from treated patients dropped sharply too at completion of irradiation and was somewhat restored by three months after irradiation. We then investigated how different cyclo-oxygenase inhibitors influenced this kind of reactivity. We used diclofenac sodium, meclofenamic acid, lysine-mono-acetylsalicylate, indomethacin as compared to ethanol, since some of these substances were dissolved in ethanol. Before irradiation all these substances substantially increased the reactivity of lymphocytes to PHA. On a molar basis, diclofenac sodium and indomethacin were most effective, but it must also be borne in mind that one can use acetylsalicylic acid in higher concentrations. The effect was much more pronounced at the completion of irradiation; and more or less unchanged three months after irradiation.

TUMOUR NECROSIS FACTOR

Tumour necrosis factor (TNF_α) is a cytokine released by macrophages and monocytes when stimulated, for example, by endotoxin. It is generally considered to be a mediator of inflammation and cytotoxicity against tumour cells and, for this reason, we were interested in *in vitro* release of TNF_α in these cancer patients after irradiation and after the addition of cyclo-oxygenase inhibitors. Since it is known that TNF_α stimulates the release of prostaglandins, we thought it would be of great interest to investigate whether irradiation affected TNF_α production.

Ten patients with breast cancer irradiated with 45 Gy, or cancer of the prostate or urinary bladder irradiated with 64 Gy, served as monocyte donors before and after treatment. Addition of indomethacin increased *in vitro* release of TNF_α from monocytes taken from the patients after radiotherapy, but not before radiotherapy. Addition of liposaccharides or endotoxin also significantly increased the release of TNF_α, both before and after radiotherapy, and the release of TNF_α after radiotherapy was significantly higher than before radiotherapy, which is of considerable interest and which has not previously been demonstrated. When we added indomethacin to our cultures we found an additional increase of release of TNF_α, both before and after radiotherapy, and the increase was higher after radiotherapy (Table 1). Irradiation-induced TNF_α release may result in an augmented production of immunosuppressive prostaglandins; this in turn should

Table 1 *Release of* TNF_α *by monocytes from irradiated cancer patients*

	Addition to cell cultures			
	None	Indomethacin	LPS[c]	LPS + indomethacin
Before radiotherapy	5.0[a]	6.2	13.3	21.2
After radiotherapy	3.1	9.7	26.9	56.3
Significance level	n.s.[b]	n.s.	$p<0.05$	$p<0.025$

[a]Concentrations of TNF_α (ng/ml) are expressed as geometric means
[b]n.s. = not significant
[c]LPS = Lipopolysaccharide
All group comparisons were made on log values using Student's t-test. LPS induced increased TNF_α release before as well as after radiotherapy ($p<0.001$) whereas indomethacin stimulated the release significantly only after therapy ($p<0.005$). Addition of indomethacin to LPS-treated cultures resulted in significantly raised levels of TNF_α before as well as after treatment ($p<0.005$ in both instances).

be expected to down-regulate TNF_{α} production through an autoregulatory circuit. Indomethacin or other cyclo-oxygenase inhibitors may prevent this hypothetical feedback inhibition and thereby increase TNF_{α} release. If these *in vitro* results are valid for the *in vivo* situation, irradiation of cancer patients might result in the release of TNF_{α}, provided that there is a concomitant activation of macrophages. Administration of a cyclo-oxygenase inhibitor could additionally stimulate the release of TNF_{α} which is endowed with antitumour activity.

In our recent experiments we demonstrated also in the same patients an increase of *in vitro* production of γ-interferon in the presence of a cyclo-oxygenase inhibitor.

The conclusion reached as a consequence of the above study was that the effects of a cyclo-oxygenase inhibitor should be examined *in vivo* in irradiated breast cancer patients, and we are planning such a study.

Most of the data in this report were presented at the Symposium on Combination Therapies, June 2, 1988 and subsequently published in *Bull N Y Acad Sci* 1989; **65** (No. 1).

DISCUSSION

Dr Lockhart: How long do you think the treatment should continue after the patients are irradiated and what dose of aspirin would you consider using, rather than indomethacin?

Dr Wasserman: We are planning studies at present which should answer this question, and we currently think that the treatment should be given for two or three months after irradiation. We have not yet decided which cyclo-oxygenase inhibitor we are going to use; it may be aspirin, diclofenac sodium, or perhaps another one.

Professor Goldstein: Have you looked at interleukin-2 in these patients?

Dr Wasserman: No we have not. We have looked for the substances I mentioned and also for interleukin-1, although I only have preliminary results for interleukin-1, showing a probable increase.

The effect of aspirin and other cyclo-oxygenase inhibitors on antitumour immunity

Jules Harris and Donald Braun

Section of Medical Oncology, Rush Cancer Center, Chicago, USA

INTRODUCTION

A number of clinical studies in the past have used aspirin as a means of altering the host-tumour balance in human cancer. One such study (1) was based on the knowledge that platelets are involved in the haematogenous spread of malignant tumours. Antiplatelet agents have inhibited the spread of tumour cells in animal model systems. However, a well-conducted clinical study (1) of adjuvant antiplatelet therapy with aspirin in colorectal cancer was negative. A more recent clinical trial (2) made the surprising observation that aspirin might act therapeutically to potentiate the clinical responses to recombinant leucocyte α-interferon in metastatic renal cell cancer. My colleagues and I were intrigued by this study; we had previously shown (3) that interferon can induce monocytes to secrete excess amounts of prostaglandins, with resultant abnormal immunoregulation. This effect could be blocked by indomethacin, an aspirin-like compound, and that suggested to us a possible explanation for how aspirin had acted in the renal cell cancer study.

Aspirin and aspirin-like compounds have profound effects on the immune system. The effect of particular interest in the context of antitumour immune mechanisms is mediated through the inhibition of prostaglandin synthetase or cyclo-oxygenase, with a resultant decrease in the secretion of prostaglandins. Cyclo-oxygenase controls the metabolic conversion of arachidonic acid from cell membrane phospholipids to prostaglandins. Aspirin-like compounds in this connection are those which, like aspirin, will inhibit the cyclo-oxygenase pathway and be potent inhibitors of prostaglandin biosynthesis. The model compound is the non-steroidal anti-inflammatory drug (NSAID) indomethacin; another such compound is piroxicam, and both indomethacin and piroxicam have been used clinically as NSAIDs.

My colleague, Dr Donald Braun, and I have recently examined the effects of prostaglandins in cancer patients and studied the biological changes in antitumour immune reactivity which may result from the use of aspirin-like compounds to block prostaglandin synthesis.

Aspirin—towards 2000, edited by G. R. Fryers, 1990; Royal Society of Medicine Services International Congress and Symposium Series No. 168, published by Royal Society of Medicine Services Limited.

PROSTAGLANDINS IN CANCER PATIENTS

There are three principal sources of prostaglandin in cancer patients. Our focus has been on the investigation of suppressor macrophages in patients with malignant disease. These suppressor macrophages exert an abnormal immunoregulatory effect on antitumour immunity through the release of excess amounts of prostaglandins. Suppressor macrophages become activated during the natural course of malignant disease and we believe that the single most important cause of immunodeficiency in cancer patients is excess release of prostaglandins by suppressor macrophages. Inhibition of prostaglandin synthesis in solid tumour cancer patient macrophages by aspirin-like drugs such as indomethacin and piroxicam will augment antitumour immunity.

A list of antitumour functions that can be augmented by prostaglandin antagonists such as cyclo-oxygenase inhibitors includes tumour-induced lymphocyte blastogenesis, cytotoxic T-cell induction, natural killer (NK) cell function, lymphokine-activated killer cell function, macrophage cytotoxicity, antitumour antibody synthesis and cytokine synthesis. Virtually all recognized antitumour immune mechanisms that have been tested have been found to be subject to modulation by amounts of prostaglandins which are produced by the suppressor monocytes of cancer patients.

Why this should be so is explained by the complex cascade of interacting cells which make up the immune system, and of the polypeptide mediator circuits that control it. The T-helper cell is the master cell of the immune system; the amplifier cell, the pivotal cell which orchestrates other immune reactivities with precision and complexity. However, it is the macrophage which functions as the sentinel cell and triggers the polypeptide mediator circuitry of the immune system through the presentation of antigen in association with interleukin-1 (IL-1), to the T-helper cell. When a resting macrophage becomes activated it will release a variety of monokines, cytokines and other factors. One of these groups is the E-type prostaglandins. The activated macrophage will at basal level release a small amount of prostaglandins and thus will regulate the immune system normally. In cancer, the activated macrophage produces an excess amount of prostaglandins and so will damp down, not only its own antitumour reactions, but all other forms of antitumour immune reactivity as well.

For the past decade Dr Braun and I have focused our attention on the suppressor macrophage in patients with malignant disease. We have studied the impact of cyclo-oxygenase products on immune function in patients with solid tumours, since these products are largely responsible for much of the immunomodulatory activity of the suppressor macrophage. These studies have confirmed that a principal source of prostaglandins in cancer patients is the suppressor macrophage. Further studies have demonstrated how this cell influences antitumour immunity in cancer patients and when, during the natural history of malignant disease, suppressor macrophages become activated (4,5). Finally, we have conducted extensive studies aimed at determining how this cell may be manipulated pharmacologically by cytotoxic chemotherapy or by prostaglandin antagonists (6). As a result of these investigations we have come to believe that the macrophage plays a key role, if not the key role, in modulating the host's antitumour immune mechanisms against cancer.

At present, most of our understanding of the usefulness of prostaglandin antagonists in modulating antitumour immunity has been based on animal models or on *in vitro* studies of peripheral blood cells in humans. However, I present below the results of studies conducted in our laboratories which were designed to measure the capacity of prostaglandin antagonists to modulate antitumour immunity in leucocytes obtained from anatomical compartments intimately associated with the tumour microenvironment. This type of study is relevant to the understanding of what actually takes place in the body at the exact site of a patient's immunological reaction against their cancer.

MACROPHAGE CYTOTOXICITY DEVELOPMENT

In our first study we investigated the development of macrophage cytotoxicity in alveolar macrophages from patients with non-small cell lung cancer. The patient population consisted of 11 individuals who were found to suffer from this disease. All patients were evaluated at the time of their initial presentation for diagnosis and staging, prior to any form of cytoreductive therapy or radiotherapy. All patients were subjected to bronchoalveolar lavage to collect alveolar macrophages and these macrophages were stimulated with 100 units/ml of γ-interferon in the presence or absence of the prostaglandin antagonist indomethacin. After overnight stimulation, the cells were washed and incubated with chromium-labelled Chang hepatoma cell targets to assess cytotoxicity. The Chang hepatoma cell is, of course, an NK-insensitive cell line. Peripheral blood monocytes from these same patients were treated in the identical manner and were analysed separately.

The results of the development of tumour cell cytotoxicity in response to γ-interferon in alveolar macrophages and peripheral blood monocytes of lung cancer patients showed first that the ability to induce macrophage cytotoxicity in alveolar macrophages was significantly reduced compared to the ability to induce cytotoxicity in peripheral blood monocytes. The mean level of cytotoxicity induced in the alveolar macrophages was significantly ($p<0.01$) less than that in the peripheral blood monocytes. The effect of indomethacin on the development of tumour cell cytotoxicity in response to γ-interferon in the alveolar macrophages and the peripheral blood monocytes of lung cancer patients was also determined. Indomethacin was not able to improve cytotoxicity significantly in the alveolar macrophages when these were considered as a group. The mean level of cytotoxicity in the alveolar macrophages in the absence of indomethacin was 3.7%; the mean level in the presence of indomethacin was 7.9%, and these differences were not significant.

However, there is a subset of patients in whom augmentation of cytotoxicity was significant. Of the 11 alveolar macrophage specimens studied, five developed a level of cytotoxicity in the presence of indomethacin which was enhanced by >100% compared to the level of cytotoxicity that developed in the absence of indomethacin. In two other specimens, 50–60% enhancement in the presence of indomethacin was observed. No augmentation of cytotoxicity was seen in the other four alveolar macrophage specimens in the presence of indomethacin. In the peripheral blood monocytes from these patients, the mean level of cytotoxicity in the absence of indomethacin was 32.3% and in the presence of indomethacin was 44.6% and this difference was significant at the $p<0.05$ level. Of the 11 individual specimens that were tested, nine demonstrated some augmentation of cytotoxicity, with four of these demonstrating >100% augmentation of cytotoxicity in the presence of indomethacin. The effect of prostaglandin antagonist treatment on peripheral blood mononuclear cells did not correlate with or predict its effect on the alveolar macrophages.

PROSTAGLANDIN ANTAGONISTS AND LAK CELL FUNCTION

In our second study we evaluated the use of prostaglandin antagonists in modulating the development of lymphokine-activated killer (LAK) cell function in the peripheral blood and tumour-infiltrating lymphocytes of patients with colon cancer. In this investigation, tumour infiltrating leucocytes were obtained from 20 primary colon tumour specimens following digestion with collagenase and DNAase and enrichment over a Ficol-Hypaque gradient. All patients were studied at the time of their initial colon tumour resection. LAK cells were induced by incubating the tumour-infiltrating leucocytes and the peripheral blood leucocytes in 500 units/ml recombinant IL-2 for three days in the presence and absence of indomethacin 2 μg/ml, and cytotoxicity was evaluated against the NK-insensitive Chang hepatoma cells.

It is clear that LAK cell induction in the tumour-infiltrating leucocytes was substantially reduced compared to the LAK induction in the peripheral blood leucocytes. The mean level of LAK activity induced in tumour-infiltrating leucocytes from the 20 colon cancer specimens was 10.2% while the mean level of LAK activity induced in the peripheral blood leucocyte cells was 34.3%, and this difference was significant at the $p<0.01$ level. In the tumour-infiltrating lymphocytes of colon cancer specimens indomethacin augmented LAK induction to a variable extent in the majority of specimens. The p value for the group approached, but did not reach, significance; $p=0.07$. Of the 20 specimens analysed, no augmentation, or minimal augmentation, was observed in 11 specimens, while >100% augmentation was observed in six specimens.

We then examined the effects of treatment with indomethacin on LAK cell induction in the peripheral blood mononuclear cells of colon cancer patients, broken down into stages B, C and D. The mean level of LAK activity in peripheral blood leucocytes from colon cancer patients was 34% in the absence of indomethacin and 39% in the presence of indomethacin. This difference was not significant when these 20 patients were considered collectively as a group. However, significant enhancement by indomethacin was observed in the subgroup of patients with Duke's stage B tumours, that is the type of tumour that was more localized than the more advanced C and D stage tumours. In those individuals, significant augmentation in the presence of indomethacin was seen in four of six cases; the mean percentage cytotoxicity for this group was 27% in the absence of indomethacin and 40% in the presence of indomethacin. This difference was significant at the $p<0.01$ level. In the patients with Duke's C tumours, significant augmentation of LAK activity by indomethacin was observed in only one of 10 cases and was not observed in any of the four Duke's stage D tumour cases.

Once again, the effect of indomethacin on LAK cell induction in the peripheral blood mononuclear cells did not correlate with the effect of indomethacin on LAK cell induction in the corresponding tumour-infiltrating leucocytes.

CONCLUSIONS (1)

From these studies we may conclude:

1. The development of tumour cell cytotoxicity in response to γ-interferon or IL-2, two biological response modifiers currently being tested for clinical cancer therapy, was significantly impaired in cells that were intimately associated with the tumour microenvironment compared to cells in the peripheral blood.

2. Prostaglandin antagonists could significantly increase the development of tumour cell cytotoxicity in tumour-associated leucocytes in a subset of the specimens tested.

3. The capacity of prostaglandin antagonists to improve the development of tumour cell cytotoxicity in tumour-associated leucocytes was not correlated with the response of peripheral blood leucocytes.

4. We believe that additional studies are needed to develop the means for utilizing prostaglandin antagonists to modulate the function of tumour-associated leucocytes *in vivo*.

IN VIVO STUDIES

Thus far, what I have described has been based on tests of cancer patient cells *in vitro*. The results have provided the theoretical basis for the use of prostaglandin antagonists to treat patients with malignant disease. However, we recently reported (7) on the actual use of prostaglandin antagonist therapy in a population of patients with cancer.

The patient population that we chose to investigate in this initial trial consisted of patients with recurrent, unresectable squamous cell carcinoma, or lymphoepithelioma of the head and neck. The rationale for this study was based on the demonstration that patients with advanced head and neck cancers have abnormal suppressor macrophages in association with immune deficiency in their peripheral blood. It was also based on anecdotal reports which suggested that prostaglandin antagonists may produce clinical responses or improve tumour control when used as neo-adjuvant therapy prior to surgery. In our study, all patients had been off previous therapy for >1 month and all presented with measurable or evaluable disease. All patients had adequate bone marrow, hepatic and renal function and a performance status of 0, 1 or 2, based on the performance status criteria of the Eastern Cooperative Oncology Group. All patients received, as prostaglandin antagonist therapy, piroxicam 20 mg, orally once daily for 30 days, together with oral antacids four times daily. A total of 10 such patients were accrued to this trial. All patients received a minimum one month of therapy with piroxicam, at which time clinical evaluation was performed in all individuals and those who had achieved disease stabilization that is, (who did not demonstrate evidence of progression) continued on treatment. Those demonstrating disease progression were removed from the study.

Overall, four patients received one month of piroxicam therapy, two additional patients received a total of two months of therapy, three additional patients received three months of therapy, and one patient received >4 months of therapy. The clinical responses that were observed in this group of patients were for the most part modest. However, five of the 10 patients did demonstrate some variable stabilization of disease, and one patient demonstrated a partial clinical response to metastatic disease in the lung.

Patient immunological monitoring which was performed during this therapy included measurements of PHA-stimulated blastogenesis, PHA-stimulated IL-2 production, NK cell function against the K562 myeloid leukaemia target cell line and an evaluation of suppressor macrophage function in the blastogenesis assay.

The results of mitogen-stimulated blastogenesis assays, prior to and following one month's piroxicam therapy are presented here. At the time of entry on therapy, 9/10 patients had a level of blastogenesis which was significantly reduced compared to normal. Following one month of therapy, blastogenesis was improved in 7/10 patients, reduced in 2/10 patients and unchanged in 1/10 patients. NK cell function in this group of individuals was also affected by one month of prostaglandin antagonist therapy. Prior to entry on therapy, 5/10 patients had significantly depressed NK cell function. At the one month assessment point significant improvement in NK cell function was observed in each of those individuals whereas a significant decline in NK cell function was seen in two other individuals, both of whom had normal levels of NK cell function prior to treatment. In the remaining individuals, NK cell function was essentially unchanged at the one month assessment point.

The effect of prostaglandin antagonist therapy on the ability of lymphocytes to produce IL-2 in response to mitogenic stimulation was also evaluated. Prostaglandin antagonist therapy did not, for the most part, affect the ability of patients' lymphocytes to produce IL-2 in response to mitogen. In fact, only 1/10 patients studied demonstrated an improvement in IL-2 production following 30 days of piroxicam treatment. However, significant improvement in the ability to respond to exogenous IL-2 *in vitro*, when this was added to PHA-stimulated cultures, was observed in the majority of patients following 30 days of piroxicam therapy. Of the 10 patients studied, significant improvement of IL-2 responsiveness was observed in 8/10 patients, with a significant decline being seen in one patient and no change in the activity being seen in the other patient.

Measurement was also undertaken of indomethacin-sensitive macrophage suppressor function in the 10 patients receiving piroxicam therapy. At the time of entry to the sudy most patients demonstrated significantly greater than normal indomethacin-sensitive macrophage suppressor function as revealed by blastogenic augmentation in the presence of indomethacin of 161% as a mean for the group. At the one-month assessment point, the four individuals who had progressive disease and who were then removed from the study continued to demonstrate elevated indomethacin-sensitive macrophage suppressor function. The six individuals with stable disease who remained on treatment showed normal macrophage suppressor function. This same pattern was seen at the two-month assessment point, at which time two additional patients developed elevated macrophage suppressor function and were also removed from the study due to progressive disease. The remaining four patients who continued to demonstrate disease stabilization continued to demonstrate normal levels of indomethacin-sensitive macrophage suppressor function. At the three-month assessment point, three individuals continued to have stable disease, but as a group demonstrated elevations in indomethacin-sensitive macrophage suppressor function. At this time, one additional individual, who was removed from the study due to disease progression, also demonstrated abnormal macrophage suppressor function. Finally, at the last assessment point, which occurred after four months of piroxicam therapy, two patients were removed from the study for disease progression and these demonstrated a modest elevation in macrophage suppressor function. The one remaining individual who continued to have stable disease had, in fact, a partial clinical regression of lung metastases and continued to demonstrate normal macrophage suppressor function.

We believe this clinical study to be remarkable. We had chosen a group of patients with advanced disease no longer responsive to cancer therapy and known to be profoundly immunosuppressed as a result of their disease and as a result also of their previous therapy with radiotherapy and chemotherapy. With an aspirin-like drug alone we had augmented some parameters of immune reactivity in these patients—including some parameters of antitumour immune reactivity. Concomitant with that we had stabilized their disease and caused, in at least one instance, some regression of disease as the result, we believe, of that augmentation of immune reactivity.

CONCLUSIONS (2)

Our conclusions for this portion of the study are:

1. Prostaglandin antagonist therapy is tolerable and is capable of potentiating some indicators of immune reactivity in the peripheral blood of treated patients.
2. Those immunological responses, which are dependent on IL-2 reactivity, were particularly sensitive to immune modulation by prostaglandin antagonist therapy.
3. Some evidence of antitumour effects were observed in these patients, with one significant tumour reduction being seen. For the most part these were modest and transient.
4. Improvement in immune function of patients treated with prostaglandin antagonist therapy was associated with the reversal of abnormal macrophage suppressor function.

SUMMARY

What I have presented demonstrates that abnormal prostaglandin biosynthesis in patients with malignant disease is a principal means whereby tumours may subvert antitumour activity and evade immunological destruction. Therefore, prostaglandin antagonists should prove useful as adjuncts for cancer therapy. This might prove to be desirable, either in postsurgical adjuvant situations where suppressor macrophages remain, or in situations where the response to biological response modifiers such as IL-2 might be limited by suppressor macrophages.

We propose that prostaglandin antagonist therapy in cancer medicine might be useful in at least the three following areas:

1. As an adjunct to biological response modifier therapy.
2. As an adjunct to cytotoxic chemotherapy.
3. As single-agent therapy in patients with abnormal suppressor macrophage function in post-treatment adjuvant settings.

Finally, continued study of prostaglandin antagonists and prostaglandin metabolism in cancer patients will provide important information about host/tumour relationships and how those relationships may be manipulated by pharmacological interventions for cancer patient benefit.

REFERENCES

(1) Lipton A, Scialla S, Harvey H, *et al.* Adjuvant antiplatelet therapy with aspirin in colorectal cancer. *J Med* 1983; **13**: 419–29.

(2) Creagan E, Buckner J, Hahn R, Richardson R, Schaid D, Kovach J. An evaluation of recombinant leukocyte A interferon with aspirin in patients with metastatic renal cell cancer. *Cancer* 1988; **61**: 1787–91.
(3) Braun DP, Harris Z, Harris JE. The effect of interferon therapy on indomethacin sensitive immunoregulation in the peripheral blood mononuclear cells of renal cell carcinoma patients. *J Biol Response Mod* 1983; **2**: 251–62.
(4) Braun DP, Nisius S, Hollinshead AC, Harris JE. Serial immune testing in surgically resected lung cancer patients. *Cancer Immunol Immunother* 1983; **15**: 114–21.
(5) Von Roenn J, Harris JE, Braun DP. Suppressor cell function in solid tumor cancer patients. *J Clin Oncol* 1987; **5**: 150–9.
(6) Braun DP, Bonomi PD, Taylor S, Harris JE. Modification of the effects of cytotoxic chemotherapy on the immune responses of cancer patients with a nonsteroidal anti-inflammatory drug, piroxicam. *J Biol Response Mod* 1987; **6**: 331–45.
(7) Braun DP, Taylor SG, Harris JE. Modulation of immunity in cancer patients by prostaglandin antagonists. *Prog Clin Biol Res* 1989; **288**: 439–49.

Aspirin and diabetes: Relevance for the prevention of microangiopathy

Paolo Pozzilli

Department of Diabetes and Immunogenetics, St Bartholomew's Hospital, London, UK and II Clinica Medice University of Rome, Italy

INTRODUCTION

There is no doubt that aspirin may have a place in diabetes, but when we talk about diabetes today we first have to discuss the role of diabetic complications in the life of the diabetic patient. Certainly, diabetic complications are the main hazard of patients living with diabetes and much has to be done in order to prevent them.

DIABETES MELLITUS AND ITS COMPLICATIONS

There are two types of diabetes mellitus. The great majority of patients suffer from non-insulin dependent diabetes mellitus (NIDDM), whereas insulin dependent diabetes mellitus (IDDM) is only found in approximately 10–15% of all patients affected by the disease. According to Grenfell and Watkins (1) diabetic nephropathy is certainly the main and most dangerous complication for patients afflicted by this disease but, when we discuss diabetes and its complications, three other disease conditions should be considered: one affects the eye and in its serious evolution becomes proliferative retinopathy; the other is neuropathy which could be both peripheral and autonomic and finally cardiac disease and peripheral vascular disease. When patients are affected by diabetic nephropathy it is very likely that they also have proliferative retinopathy, neuropathy and other diseases, and this is true for both types of diabetes; however we should say that patients with NIDDM tend to suffer more of macrovascular than microvascular disease, while the converse is typical of patients with IDDM.

Diabetic nephropathy is the main hazard, as can be seen in three prospective studies, the UK study, the Steno Memorial Hospital study in Denmark, and the Joslin Clinic study in Boston (see (1)). Renal failure is the main cause of death in patients who have been affected by long standing diabetes. The percentages are very similar in the three studies, >50% of diabetic patients dying of renal failure, whereas cardiovascular disease is probably less frequent because these patients die of renal failure first.

But another complication, which is perhaps not taken into consideration so much, is autonomic neuropathy. One study performed by Ewing and his

Aspirin—towards 2000, edited by G. R. Fryers, 1990; Royal Society of Medicine Services International Congress and Symposium Series No. 168, published by Royal Society of Medicine Services Limited.

collaborators (2), showed that patients with diabetes who suffer autonomic neuropathy tend to have a strikingly lower survival rate than patients affected by diabetes without autonomic neuropathy, and by five years, approximately 50% of these patients die of diseases that could be related to the development of autonomic neuropathy. It is obvious that, because this is a slowly progressive disease, attempts must be made in order to slow down its development.

Considering diabetic nephropathy and the three main variables associated with it—glomerular filtration rate, albumin excretion rate and kidney volume—three main therapies are considered today. These are: antihypertensive treatment, strict glycaemic control, and a low protein diet. The latter may affect the glomerular filtration rate and this may have a positive effect on the evolution of diabetic nephropathy, but I would like to stress that strict glycaemic control is the main goal in patients with diabetes, together with the low protein diet. There is no doubt that in Europe, and in particular in the southern part where the protein content in the diet is lower than in northern Europe, diabetic nephropathy appears to be less frequent; interestingly amongst patients admitted to dialysis centres in Southern Europe there are fewer diabetic patients compared with Northern Europe (3).

ASPIRIN AND INSULIN

It has been known since the beginning of this century that aspirin could increase insulin secretion, but unfortunately for aspirin, this was noted at about the time when insulin was discovered and, therefore, aspirin was not taken into consideration for treatment of diabetes as perhaps it might otherwise have been. Dr Micossi in Milan and Professor Foa in Detroit investigated in a modern fashion the role that aspirin may have on the dynamics of insulin secretion. They showed that a high dose of aspirin can stimulate insulin and glucagon secretion and increase the glucose tolerance, both in normal and in diabetic subjects; however, this effect was observed only at very high doses (more than 2 g of aspirin).

ASPIRIN AND NON-ENZYMIC GLYCATION

I wish to examine the possible effect that aspirin may have on the non-enzymic glycation induced by high concentrations of glucose. Many have attempted to identify a common pathway to the development of diabetic complications; it is well known that in diabetes the eye, the kidney, the heart, the tissues in general may be exposed to increased glycosylation and, therefore, if we can block, or at least reduce, non-enzymic glycation, we may interfere with a common pathway that is increased in diabetes. Therefore, in seeking a role for aspirin in diabetes, three different possible targets should be considered: the metabolic target, the vascular target and the target represented by the circulating and structural proteins.

The stimulation of insulin secretion and the improvement of glucose tolerance induced by aspirin in patients with NIDDM are not reviewed here. Another aspect is the well-known inhibition of the cyclo-oxygenase system induced by aspirin, and in this context this drug may have in diabetes the same role of protection from cardiovascular disease shown in normal subjects. A third new aspect which deserves attention is the inhibition of the protein non-enzymic glycation, a mechanism playing an important role in the development of diabetic complications.

When glucose is present in high concentrations as may occur in diabetes, it reacts with the free amino-acid group to form a labile chemical entity, the Schiff's base, which undergoes a slow rearrangement and ends in the appearance of a more stable compound, the Amadori product. In structural long-lived proteins such as collagen, myelin and cristallin, the Amadori products undergo a further series of dehydration which results in the appearance of stable glycation end products. One of these glycated proteins is glycosylated haemoglobin (HbA_1), whose measurement is well known for the evaluation of metabolic control.

Circulating proteins include, among others, haemoglobin, albumin, globulin fractions and serum lipoproteins. If the content of glucose in a protein is increased, its properties may change also. For instance, by increasing the amount of HbA_1, one can increase the affinity for oxygen and if glycosylation of a lipoprotein is augmented there is a modification in the specificity of the low density lipoprotein receptor. Perhaps this could be one mechanism responsible for atherogenesis. The glomerular basement membrane which is particularly important in diabetes as it may become thickened if glycosylated, is characterized by an abnormal cross-linking with possible alteration of the structure and of the filtration properties. This might be one of the mechanisms responsible for the deterioration of renal function in diabetes. Also, the increased glycosylation of the structural proteins in the aorta and the coronary arteries has been suggested to explain the higher frequency of heart disease in diabetic patients. Even the protein of crystallin can be glycosylated and this process may favour the insurgence of cataract in diabetes.

Data obtained at post mortem by investigating several tissues (aorta, coronary artery, peripheral nerve, lung connective tissue and glomerular basement membrane) indicate that the amount of glucose present in these tissues is increased in patients with diabetes. Furthermore, other proteins such as albumin, α_1-, α_2-, β- and γ-globulin, and fibrinogen in diabetic patients are glycosylated in higher amounts than in normal subjects. The question therefore is, what is the relationship between these data and the insurgence of diabetic complications? A positive correlation was observed between the amount of non-enzymic glycation of the aortic tissue in patients with diabetes and the development of diabetic complications. Based on these findings, we have investigated *in vitro* the effect that aspirin may have on non-enzymic glycation (4). Different proteins, including glomerular basement membrane, have been studied. We have demonstrated an effect of aspirin on *in vitro* non-enzymic glycation of human albumin and fibrinogen. Thus, by increasing the concentration of glucose, the amount of glycosylated protein was also increased. The effect of glucose concentration was highly significant, and the addition of aspirin to the medium was capable of reducing the non-enzymic glycation of tested proteins. Aspirin was added in concentrations which were 1/10 of glucose varying from 5 to 100 mmol/l. Only at concentrations >25 mmol/l glucose, was aspirin effective. So, at least *in vitro*, and at rather high concentrations, aspirin inhibits this pathway.

Clinical studies are necessary to evaluate whether aspirin may be a useful adjunct to good metabolic control in reducing non-enzymic glycation and preventing diabetic complications. In an open study which began in 1984 (5) aspirin at 500 mg daily was given to 39 patients with NIDDM (in addition to antidiabetic therapy) and the effect of this regimen on the progression of microalbuminuria and retinopathy was evaluated. After three years there was a slight but not significant decrease in microalbuminuria in the aspirin treated group compared to the control group; as far as retinopathy is concerned, in the course of 3.5 years follow-up there was no difference in the appearance of retinal lesions in patients treated with aspirin and the control group. A multicentre randomized controlled trial presented elsewhere in this book showed that aspirin at 330 mg daily + dipyridamole is capable of reducing the evolution of microaneurisms in early diabetic retinopathy.

Finally, the European Community has this year launched the Eurodiab project, an EEC-wide concerted approach to diabetes, involving studies on pathogenesis, complications and education. In view of the present results the effect of aspirin in controlling the spread of diabetic late complications deserves more attention in the future, in the hope that this compound may help to prevent the devastating effects of a chronic disease such as diabetes.

REFERENCES

(1) Grenfell A, Watkins PJ. Clinical diabetic nephropathy: natural history and complications. *Clin Endocrinol Metab* 1986; **15**: 783–806.
(2) Ewing DJ, Campbell IW, Clarke BF. The natural history of diabetic autonomic neuropathy. *Quart J Med* 1980; **193**: 95–108.
(3) Pozzilli P, Corcos A, Visalli N, Andreani D. Diabetic patients attending dialysis centres in Central Italy. *J Diabetic Complications* 1987; **2**: 1–4.
(4) Sensi M, Bruno MR, Pozzilli P. *In vitro* inhibition of non-enzymatic glycosylation induced by aspirin. *Med Sci Res* 1987; **15**: 99–100.
(5) Corcos A, Colletti F, Tarentini M, *et al.* Treatment of Type 2 diabetes with aspirin: effect on metabolic control. In: Crepaldi G, Cunha Vas JG, Fedele D, Mogensen CE, Ward JD, eds. *Microvascular and neurological complications of diabetes*. Fidia Research Series No. 10. New York, Berlin: Springer Verlag, 1987.

Effect of aspirin in early diabetic retinopathy: A multicentre, randomized, controlled clinical trial

Gerard Slama

Department of Diabetes, Hotel-Dieu Hospital, Paris, France

INTRODUCTION

This presentation will discuss the results of the Dipyridamole, Aspirin, Microaneurysm And Diabetes (DAMAD) study (1) which compared the effect of aspirin, or aspirin plus another platelet aggregation inhibitor, dipyridamole, in early diabetic retinopathy. This was a multicentre, double-blind, randomized, controlled clinical trial.

There was one co-ordinating centre in Paris, led by Dr Evelyn Eschwege, two haematology centres, one in the Hotel-Dieu Hospital in Paris and the other in Edinburgh, and four clinical centres, one in the Hotel-Dieu Hospital, Paris, another at Sainte-Louis Hospital, Paris, one in University Hospital, Cardiff and the other at the Hammersmith Hospital, London.

PROTOCOL

The protocol was designed in 1976, which explains why we chose an aspirin dosage of 1 g: at that time there was no evidence to guide us otherwise. The protocol allowed for a patient selection period in the four centres, a run-in period where the patients were given placebo for one month, then all elected patients who were willing to participate were randomized between three groups: one a placebo group, one with aspirin and one aspirin plus dipyridamole. All received one tablet three times a day, either 1/3 g aspirin, 1/3 g aspirin plus 75 mg dipyridamole, or a matching placebo. They were then followed on an outpatient clinic basis every four months during the three years of follow-up. On a clinical basis the physician had to classify seven types of fundus modification like hard exudate, soft exudate, macular oedema, other macular lesions, neovascularization and other fundus complications, and on this basis the doctors had to say whether there was improvement, stabilization or worsening of the appearance of the fundus. The appearance of the fundus deteriorated somewhat in some patients, but with no significant difference between placebo, aspirin or aspirin plus dipyridamole on this clinical criterion.

Aspirin—towards 2000, edited by G. R. Fryers, 1990; Royal Society of Medicine Services International Congress and Symposium Series No. 168, published by Royal Society of Medicine Services Limited.

The inclusion criteria were as follows:
—Either Type 1 or Type 2 diabetes mellitus (we tried to provide equal numbers of each type)
—Age 17–67 years
—No other diseases present such as abnormal ECG, elevated blood pressure
—Frankly diabetic with a fasting blood glucose >6 mmol/l or a 2 h post-prandial blood glucose >10 mmol/l.
—>5 microaneurysms in the central part of the fundus.
—No other disease contraindicating either aspirin or dipyridamole present.

PATIENTS AND METHODS

More than 10 000 patients were screened and only 778 went to angiography, of whom only 475 were eventually randomized, out of whom 420 completed the whole study. Some 8% of patients were lost to follow-up, which is not a bad result for such a long trial.

Compliance was assessed on the number of visits attended or missed, secondly on the inhibition with arachidonic acid of platelet aggregation, and third (in one centre) by the tablet count. Seventy-five per cent of patients attended all planned visits, and 85% attended the annual visit which was the most important one each year, which is also satisfactory.

On metabolic criteria, we believe that 9% of the patients on placebo were also probably taking drugs containing aspirin without the knowledge of the doctor, as indicated by our tests. Eleven per cent of the patients supposed to take aspirin had normal platelet aggregation at the time of the test which means that, at least for the few days preceding the blood sampling, they were not taking the drug.

The judgment criteria were:
—Ophthalmoscopy performed by clinical ophthalmologists
—Angiography read by trained technicians without either knowledge of the conclusion or the type of treatment taken.

RESULTS

The placebo, aspirin and combination therapy groups were comparable. The insulin-treated group had normal body weight, with mean fasting plasma glucose >170 mg and mean postprandial glucose >180 mg, and normal blood pressure. The non-insulin treated patients were slightly overweight and less hyperglycaemic than the insulin-treated patients.

The 41 patients who did not complete the study did not exhibit different characteristics from the group completing the study, but there were significantly fewer patients lost to follow-up in the aspirin group than in the placebo and aspirin plus dipyridamole groups. We observed eight deaths during the three-year study: four deaths in the placebo-treated group and four deaths in the aspirin or aspirin plus dipyridamole groups; three myocardial infarctions in the placebo group and four in the aspirin-treated group, with no statistical difference on this very small number of deaths.

We were obliged to undertake some photocoagulation of the retina during the study but no more in the placebo than in either of the two active groups.

We were also obliged to discontinue drug treatment of some patients during the three years, with the same number of discontinuations in each group, but gastrointestinal symptoms were seven times more frequent in the two actively treated groups than in the placebo group, which is not really surprising, particularly with the high dose of aspirin used. There were many other causes for discontinuing the treatment, such as pregnancy, vomiting or gastritis.

Most importantly, we tried to determine the number of definite unequivocal microaneurysms at entry. No statistically significant difference at entry was found in NID diabetics, even though in the placebo group there was a mean of 3.7 microaneurysms, whereas there were 6.5 in the aspirin-treated group. Likewise, in ID diabetics there was no significant difference at baseline concerning the number of definite microaneurysms in the fundus.

At the end of the study the progression of the number of microaneurysms was significantly lower in the aspirin and aspirin-plus-dipyridamole groups altogether as compared with the placebo group. Comparing the three groups there is no significant difference, but when we put together the group with aspirin and the group receiving aspirin plus dipyridamole there is a highly significant difference between this group and the placebo group (result being much better in the other group). This effect is significant in both Type 1 (ID) and Type 2 (NID) diabetes.

CONCLUSIONS

In this long-lasting study, aspirin, either alone or in combination with dipyridamole, was able to retard the progression of retinopathy in early diabetic retinopathy. The clinical improvement was too small for an unequivocal statement that all such patients should be treated with aspirin, but this study adds weight to others which have indicated that it is probably worth while to give aspirin to diabetic patients at the very beginning, almost as primary prevention of diabetic retinopathy.

REFERENCE

(1) Dipyridamole, Aspirin, Microaneurysm and Diabetes (DAMAD) Study Group. The effect of aspirin alone and aspirin plus dipyridamole in early diabetic retinopathy by the DAMAD study group. *Diabetes* 1989; **38**: 491–6.

DISCUSSION

Dr Pozzilli: What was the level of HbA_1 in the groups that received aspirin plus dipyridamole, compared with the group that received placebo?

Dr Slama: There was no significant difference in terms of HbA_{1c} between the three groups initially, neither was there a difference between the three groups at the end of three years' study. However, there was a significant improvement, at least in the first year, between baseline and post-treatment, which means that all patients improved when entering the study, a phenomenon which is well known. However, it does not appear that aspirin has a specific impact on HbA_{1c} in this study.

Professor Cotlier: As an ophthalmologist I would like to congratulate Dr Slama for this excellent study. It tackles one of the most difficult parts of diabetic retinopathy, trying to go over the initial phase, the stage that may take three, five or more years to develop, the early stages of retinopathy. That is very courageous, I do not know of anybody who has tried to tackle the very early phase as thoroughly as you have done, and have such a degree of control over the entire population with a large number of patients, taking into consideration all the variety of things that you have done. I am very pleased to say your study meets very high scientific standards.

There is a component of platelet aggregation in the formation of diabetic retinopathy that has been postulated many times but never really been demonstrated except that some patients with known diabetic retinopathy who have been tested by aggregometry seem to have a much greater aggregation of platelets. If this population has already developed diabetic retinopathy you could take them at a later stage and then try to do a trial with aspirin. It might last a shorter time but would give you a more definite answer in the stage of progression, because you are trying at a very early stage when the disease moves rather slowly.

Dr Slama: We will not lose these patients to follow-up of course, but we would take 10 more years to report the results. You are right that a more advanced retinopathy would have been a better model in which to study the problem, but at that time we did not have the tool to measure blindly the progression on angiography, we needed a measurement criterion and now we have a computerized model. Neovascularization does not need any computer, but areas of non-perfusion do, for it is easy to say they are present but not easy to compare and calculate.

Dr Lockhart: What criteria did you use to reduce the thousands of patients down to 700 patients to undergo angiography?

Dr Slama: When I said that more than 10 000 patients were screened, a technician made the decision whether every diabetic patient was eligible for the study. Some were not, due to age, associated illness, very advanced retinopathy, for example, or myocardial infarction in their history. This is the reason why only 500 met the criteria. In our centres where only more complicated patients were followed, very few met the criteria of very early retinopathy with no associated illness.

Dr Pozzilli: Dr Slama started with eight microaneurysms per eye in patients with NIDDM and 3.7 in the placebo control group, and he ended with one aneurysm per eye in the placebo control group. This is a remarkable result, despite the fact that these were just patients with diabetes who were followed up for such a long period of time. I think that the message would be that, if you control your diabetic patient well at the beginning of the disease, or when early retinopathy develops, you can protect these patients from the development of severe retinopathy. If you also treat them with aspirin, according to Dr Slama's data, you may even improve the result. That is the most important message, that metabolic control is probably the key to preventing complications of the disease.

Dr Fryers: Are we looking here at a prostaglandin mechanism or is this a link to inhibition of glycosylation, or some other?

Dr Slama: I cannot answer the question because the trial was undertaken on a pragmatic rather than an explicative basis. We measured parameters, but we are not able to say through which mechanism the results were mainly achieved.

Dr Pozzilli: We can only speculate that, if metabolic control is relevant in reducing the development of diabetic complications, this has something to do with the glycosylation of proteins.

Dr Fryers: I was speculating similarly, because if it was a prostaglandin mechanism, one would expect to find increased prostaglandins in the condition if we do not treat it with aspirin. Aspirin would only work to suppress that which was being produced, and I wondered if any of these complications had ever been seen, for instance, in chronic inflammations, where you would expect to have quite high levels of prostaglandins. My own reflection was probably not, but if it is a glycosylation of proteins, do we know much about the dosage that is necessary to be effective on glycosylating proteins? You have produced some *in vitro* figures, Dr Pozzilli, but do we know in humans what is the required dose?

Dr Pozzilli: No, we have no idea what dose of aspirin would be required *in vivo* for such an effect and we also have to consider that glycosylation is a process which affects proteins that have different life spans. Thus, a protein like the lens has a very long life, whereas other proteins have a very short life. Glycosylation of such proteins depends upon the length of poor metabolic control. It is well known that patients who are poorly controlled tend to develop diabetic complications over a period of time, whereas patients who are well controlled do not. Therefore, when the issue of aspirin dose is considered, we should also take well into account the protein we are looking at and the degree of metabolic control.

Dr Fryers: Do we know when we acetylate the protein (and presumably that is the mechanism by which you stop it glycosylating) whether the acetyl group is linking on to the same point as that to which glucose would link?

Dr Pozzilli: Yes, it appears to be the same point.

Dr Fryers: In which case the final point of my argument is that it would be specifically aspirin and not a non-steroidal anti-inflammatory effect to reduce non-enzymic glycation of proteins.

Dr Pozzilli: I agree with your comment.

Professor de Gaetano: What were the confidence limits of your results? I noticed a very large standard deviation of your means, 0.5 ± 5, so it seems that these average values are very widely scattered.

Dr Slama: The confidence limit chosen was α-risk 0.05 and β-risk 0.005, and the levels of significance were also 0.05, so even though there was a scatter of results, those were significant in some respects. It might be that for some parameters we did not find a significant difference due to that, but when you find it, it means that they exist.

Dr Harding: In relation to the discussion on glycation, it has been shown that aspirin can decrease the glycation of retinal basement membrane, so it might be relevant in retinopathy. The less good news is that it has also been shown, for example, that ibuprofen can inhibit glycation just as aspirin does and obviously not by acetylation.

Dr Pozzilli: Other studies have been carried out using glomerular basement membrane and similar results have been obtained with isolated human glomerular basement membrane and aspirin, suggesting that even a structural protein like the basement membrane can be in some way modified in its capacity to be glycosylated.

Dr Petersen-Braun: If you repeated the study you just have completed, what dose of aspirin would you choose? Would you still choose 1 g?

Dr Slama: With aspirin 1 g such results were observed. I would not like to extend this conclusion to other dosages. Subjectively I would tend to say that 300 mg would be nice, but I really have no scientific grounds for saying that.

Dr Fryers: If I may add to that, if acetylation is the mechanism, then giving a large dose of a quickly absorbed form of aspirin would be the way to get it there and not several small doses scattered throughout the day, so there is a pharmacokinetic question too, which will depend on the mechanism of action.

Dr Slama: But, conversely, a large dose might increase the side-effects.

Dr Fryers: It certainly would tend to do so.

Dr Lockhart: Dr Slama, you may be aware of the National Eye Institute study in the USA which will conclude at the end of this year, and which is also looking at diabetic retinopathy over a 10-year span, although I am not sure how long the follow-up is. I believe that, again, the aspirin dose is 1×325 mg tablet three times daily, so if the study does find similar results we will not know what the dose should be, except we will know that 1 g daily will be the dose at this point in time—we may never get another dose, though.

Clinical and epidemiological aspects of Reye's syndrome

John F. T. Glasgow and Raymond Moore

Department of Child Health, The Queen's University of Belfast, Belfast, UK

CHRONOLOGY

Perhaps the first description of a group of children with Reye's syndrome (RS) was as long ago as 1929 by the late Lord Brain and colleagues (1). Single case reports of likely cases were reported during the next 30 years or so, but it was not until 1963 that the two definitive papers appeared, one from Australia by R. D. K. Reye and colleagues (2) and the other from North Carolina by G. M. Johnson and colleagues (3). These described a total of 36 children, the majority of whom died or sustained severe, permanent neurological damage and were thought to define a novel clinico-pathological entity.

My interest was awakened in 1967 when an unconscious child was admitted to the Royal Belfast Hospital for Sick Children. Unfortunately she rapidly succumbed and at autopsy we identified in the stomach contents a variety of commercial paint thinners, chemical analysis of which mirrored that frequently used in a near-by car bodywork spraying firm (4).

Another UK milestone was the establishment in 1976 (to 1979) of the National Childhood Encephalopathy Study in England, Scotland and Wales. This was an epidemiological study of children under three years of age with acute neurological disorders, of which 37 fulfilled the diagnostic criteria of RS (5). As a result it became apparent that much more information was required and on 1 August 1981 the British Reye's Syndrome Surveillance Scheme (BRSSS) commenced. This was (at first) a voluntary (passive) reporting scheme and sought to monitor cases throughout the UK and the Republic of Ireland. A change to *active* ascertainment, using monthly prompt cards sent to all paediatricians, was introduced in July 1986 when the British Paediatric Surveillance Unit was established. Information from these schemes (1.8.1981–31.7.1988, 422 cases (6) and our own personal experience of 57 cases, since 1.1.1979), has provided the clinical information upon which this paper is based (7).

It had already been recognized by paediatric neurologists that *acute encephalopathy* in childhood was a formidable clinical problem. It tended to strike without warning following an otherwise relatively trivial respiratory or gastrointestinal infection and often proved rapidly fatal. It was appreciated that

Aspirin—towards 2000, edited by G. R. Fryers, 1990; Royal Society of Medicine Services International Congress and Symposium Series No. 168, published by Royal Society of Medicine Services Limited.

should the child survive, they may be left with permanent neurological damage; recovery, however, was possible. This description given in 1961 by Dodge and colleagues (8) came two years before the now classic paper by Reye and colleagues (2).

DIAGNOSTIC CRITERIA

Classical RS is a biphasic illness, in that neurological deterioration occurs several (in N. Ireland three) days after an otherwise trivial, probably viral, prodrome. The neurological deterioration is usually heralded by repeated vomiting, sometimes of altered blood, and the child, who is most often of preschool age (median age in UK 15 months) (2,6,7) declines into unconsciousness, sometimes associated with seizures, and, unless effective therapy is initiated promptly, death or serious handicap will ensue.

Suggestive biochemical features are elevation of the blood ammonia, the aspartate or alanine aminotransferases to greater than three times the upper limit for the laboratory. Crucially, there must not be *another more reasonable explanation for the child's illness*. Much depends upon the biochemical sophistication upon which an individual clinician can call and with what vigour the diagnosis of an inborn error of metabolism (IEM) is pursued (see below). The Third Annual Report of the British Paediatric Surveillance Unit points out, however, that relatively few of the cases reported in recent years have had the necessary, detailed, diagnostic studies done, in spite of the fact that a diagnosis of IEM is more likely today than that of 'true' (or classical) RS (see below) (6).

The diagnosis is *confirmed* by liver biopsy (or autopsy) when a very heavy, microvesicular, panlobular, fatty infiltration is found. There are also characteristic mitochondrial changes on electron microscopy. These consist of large, pleomorphic mitochondria which also show disruption of the cristae and loss of the dense body. This appears to be an acute and universal finding, which tends to resolve very rapidly if the patient improves (9). The changes appear to be quite distinct from those found in the IEMs which can mimic some of the clinical and biochemical features of RS (see p. 75). Incidentally they are also distinct from those seen in acute salicylate intoxication.

A certain degree of clinical heterogeneity in the presentation of RS has been reported. In addition to the *classical* case described above, *milder* examples have been recognized; for instance a patient recovering from a trivial, pyrexial illness developed mild vomiting associated with an elevation of the serum transaminases. Following intravenous glucose there was a rapid improvement (10). At the other extreme, 10% of our patients presented in a fulminant way, following an extremely short prodrome, with very rapid deterioration in the level of consciousness—similar to so-called, 'near miss sudden infant death syndrome'. The latter were all very young and all were profoundly hypoglycaemic. In the group (of 57) as a whole a low blood glucose occurred in 47%, while all showed a prolonged prothrombin time.

EPIDEMIOLOGY

In Northern Ireland (population 1.6 million) since 1979 we have treated 57 patients. Mean annual incidence (1979/87) has been higher than in any other region of the UK—1.9 per 100 000 children <16 years of age (11), with a peak in 1984

Table 1 *Reye's syndrome in Northern Ireland 1979–87*

Year	No. of cases (and incidence[a])	
1979	2 (0.5)	likely incomplete ascertainment
1980	7 (1.6)	
1981	3 (0.7)	
1982	9 (2.1)	
1983	12 (2.8)	
1984	14 (3.3)	
1985	9 (2.1)	
1986	1 (0.2)	
1987	0 (0)	

[a]per 100 000 under 16 years of age.

of 3.3/100 000 (12) (Table 1). In contrast to patients reported from North America, UK cases have been very young (see above) and have occurred sporadically. In N. Ireland we could detect no space : time clustering (13) nor in the UK as a whole has there been an association with outbreaks of influenza or varicella.

MANAGEMENT AND OUTCOME

Management should be carried out by a multidisciplinary team in a paediatric intensive therapy unit, employing a combination of direct intracranial pressure monitoring together with strenuous measures to reduce cerebral oedema, which is the principal cause of morbidity and mortality (14).

AETIOLOGY AND PATHOGENESIS

This is a potential minefield and has proved a difficult area to investigate convincingly. Reye made reference to the fact that the appearance and clinical presentation of RS were reminiscent of vomiting sickness of Jamaica, which is attributed to hypoglycin poisoning from eating unripe ackee fruit (9). Studies in north-east Thailand in the 1970s investigated the association of a similar, but perhaps slightly different, encephalopathy with the eating of aflatoxin-contaminated foods. Studies in Nova Scotia investigated an association with crop-spraying against bud worm. The emulsifiers and the actual sprays themselves have each been suggested as aetiological factors. Yet a further agent—Margosa oil, ingested in excess amounts—has been reported from Malaysia to result in similar clinical features. Recently a number of plausible, biochemical mechanisms which may be involved in pathogenesis were reviewed (13).

Today, however, it is appreciated that a number of IEMs can mimic RS. Hence it is vital to carry out the sorts of investigations which we have recently established in our laboratory and which Dr Priscille Divry from Lyon details in her paper (p. 75).

Drug ingestion and Reye's syndrome

The question of RS being linked to drug ingestion has been investigated in the US in a series of epidemiological, case-control studies published in the early 1980s (16–18). Exposure to aspirin was specifically investigated by interviews carried out either in the admitting hospital in RS cases, or in the patient's home in the case of controls. These studies sought to show that there was an association between the taking of aspirin during the prodrome and the development of the syndrome. However, following the release of the raw data to independent assessors, called in by the aspirin manufacturers, a number of design biases were revealed. Perhaps the most important of these was selection bias. In particular, the RS cases and the controls were not matched for the degree of illness. Thus the RS cases, who were probably the more ill, might have been more likely to have been given aspirin. Other forms of bias, recently reviewed by Susan Hall (19) (recall bias, data collection bias, protopathic bias and categorization bias) were also present. These biases have called these findings into question. They may also have created an atmosphere which biased future epidemiological research, perhaps to the extent that some paediatricians may have considered the diagnosis of RS *only* when aspirin had been given (i.e. further selection bias).

In spite of considerable criticism of these findings, two subsequent studies conducted by the US Public Health Laboratory Service, confirmed an association between aspirin and RS (20,21). In spite of strenuous efforts to exclude bias, some, particularly in relation to recall and categorization, were still present. Moreover, liver biopsy confirmation in these studies of RS was also scanty. Nevertheless a very strong association with prodromal aspirin use was still present, the relative risk of developing RS, if aspirin had been given, being extremely high (16 and 26 in the pilot and main studies). The more recently published of these contained only 27 patients with RS stage II or deeper, perhaps reflecting the difficulty in recruiting more patients. A very recent multicentre study coordinated by workers at Yale was designed in a particular critical manner. Researchers went to great lengths to exclude any degree of bias, but still reported a highly significant association between RS and aspirin (22). Interestingly, in this most convincing of comparisons, there was also a dose related effect. Summary findings of all these studies are shown in Table 2. A small Japanese study however, remains the only investigation in which this association could not be confirmed (23).

The UK Risk Factor Study conducted by Hall and colleagues (24) also found an association between the taking of pre-admission aspirin and the development of RS. This study, based upon 106 BRSSS cases reported between 1981–84 was

Table 2 *Summary of epidemiological studies linking Reye's Syndrome with aspirin*

	Exposure aspirin			Exposure paracetamol		
Study	Cases (%)	Controls (%)	*p*	Controls (%)	Cases (%)	*p*
Arizona 1978	7/7(100)	8/16(50)	<0.05	6/16(38)	1/7(14)	NS
Michigan 1980	24/25(96)	30/46(65)	<0.002	16/46(35)	1/25(4)	<0.005
Michigan 1980–81	12/12(100)	13/29(45)	<0.002	16/29(55)	0/12(0)	<0.005
Ohio 1978–80	94/97(97)	110/156(71)	<0.001[a]	52/156(33)	17/97(16)	<0.01
US PHS 1984 (pilot)	28/30(93)	65/145(46)	<0.001[c]	97/145(67)	8/30(27)	<0.001
US PHS 1985–86 (Main)	26/27(96)	45/140(32)	<0.001[d]			
Yale Multicentre Study 1986–87	21/24(88)	8/48(17)[b]		34/48(71)	9/24(38)	

[a]Relative risk 11.5
[b]Relative risk 35
[c]Relative risk 16.1
[d]Relative risk 26.0

designed initially as a 'fishing expedition', but when it was found, rather unexpectedly, that 63/106 patients had received prior aspirin therapy, it was considered necessary to collect *comparison data* on pre-admission drug usage in non-RS children. Two comparison groups of 185 febrile, hospital admissions were recruited (during 1985 and early 1986), one in South London, the other in Belfast. These comparison groups should not be regarded as 'control patients', since they were not matched for age, sex, geography or year of inclusion; this was not therefore a case-control study. Nonetheless, the findings of this comparison are interesting in that they supported those of the earlier US studies.

Although similar overall proportions of cases and comparison patients had received antipyretics, 63/106 (59%) of cases and 48/185 (26%) comparison patients were given aspirin ($p<0.00015$). (There was also found to be an excess exposure to aspirin in children under five years of age.) Conversely, 25% of cases had been given paracetamol compared to 49% of comparison patients ($p=0.00015$). Separate analyses within the Northern Ireland and London groups also showed a case-comparison difference. Moreover, Belfast *comparison patients* had received aspirin significantly more frequently than those in London ($p=0.0014$). This greater *overall* use of aspirin in Northern Ireland might have been a contributory factor to the much higher incidence of RS in that part of the UK.

Because of the non-specificity of the RS diagnostic criteria, Dr Hall developed the 'Reye score'. Each clinical, biochemical or pathological feature was arbitrarily allotted one point. Accordingly scores could range up to 17, higher scores being associated with classical cases while those with low scores revealed diagnostic uncertainty. This analysis also showed a strong association between the 'Reye score' and the likelihood of the patient having received an antipyretic. Analysis by type of medication, showed a highly significant correlation between aspirin exposure and the score (trend $p=0.0001$), in contrast to that for paracetamol ($p=0.07$). This was further evidence that the association between the classical case and prodromal aspirin medication was extremely strong.

Pattern of events since June 1986

Taking all of this evidence together, the Committee on Safety of Medicines (CSM), recommended in 1986 that aspirin should not be given to children aged under 12 years, except on medical advice (25). They concluded that aspirin may be a contributory factor in causing *some* cases of RS. The CSM Chairman wrote to all doctors, dentists and pharmacists advising them of these opinions and stating that paediatric aspirin preparations would be withdrawn from sale. Subsequently, there was a public information campaign and labelling changes. In any case, prior to this announcement, the UK aspirin manufacturers had requested that all children's aspirin preparations be removed from the shelves of retail outlets.

Table 3 *Clinical staging (Modified Lovejoy Staging) in relation to outcome*

Stage	Patients	Full recovery (%)
1	7	7 (100)
2	19	17 (90)
3	24	16 (67)
4	6	2 (33)

$\chi^2=10.7$; $p=0.01$.

Since then, the number of cases of RS reported to BRSSS has declined, from a peak of 79 in 1983/84 to 27 in 1988/89 (6). It is our impression that many of these cases are also less characteristic of RS (possibly with a lower 'Reye score'—although specific data on this are not yet available) than those being reported in the early 1980s. The decline in case numbers has been most dramatic in Northern Ireland (but might possibly have begun before 1986) (12) (Table 3). A similar reduction in reported cases has been described in the US where this has apparently closely paralleled that in sales of children's aspirin (26,27).

Finally an as yet unpublished study, of 101 febrile (non-RS) children being admitted to hospital during 1988 and early 1989, 53 in Belfast and 48 in London (from the same centres which participated in the earlier comparison study), showed that only two children, one in each centre, had been given aspirin prior to admission. Children were therefore, 17 times *less* likely to have received aspirin in 1988/89 than in 1985/86 (28). The public education campaign to discourage the use of aspirin in febrile children has succeeded only partially, however, since 40% of Belfast parents and 27% of London parents had heard of RS, while much smaller percentages (23% and 15%, respectively) knew of its association with aspirin.

In our opinion therefore, the evidence outlined above seems to suggest that it is likely that aspirin has been causative in some (classical) cases of RS.

SUMMARY

RS is a serious, acute encephalopathy of childhood, the diagnosis of which presents clinical difficulty and is largely a matter of careful exclusion, particularly of inborn errors of metabolism. Early clinical recognition and prompt management are crucial if mortality and morbidity are to be reduced. UK data has confirmed US findings that there is an association between RS and the use of pre-admission aspirin.

N. Ireland has a well worked-out central referral policy for very ill children requiring intensive therapy which has greatly helped case ascertainment and reporting. Prior to 1986 we had the highest UK incidence of RS combined with significantly greater use of aspirin among both cases and (non-RS) febrile children than in similar groups in London. This association together with a 17-fold reduction in the use of childhood aspirin in 1988/89 linked to the more recent striking decline in the numbers of actively reported cases, is we believe, among the more convincing evidence that there is a causal link between aspirin medication and RS.

REFERENCES

(1) Brain WR, Turnbull HM. Acute meningoencephalomyelitis of childhood. *Lancet* 1929; **i**: 221–7.

(2) Reye RDK, Morgan G, Baral J. Encephalopathy and fatty degeneration of the viscera: a disease entity in childhood. *Lancet* 1963; **ii**: 749–52.

(3) Johnson GM, Scurletis TD, Carrol MB. A study of 16 fatal cases of encephalitis-like disease in North Carolina children. *N Carolina Med J* 1963; **24**: 464–73.

(4) Glasgow JFT, Ferris JAJ. Encephalopathy and fatty infiltration of probable toxic aetiology. *Lancet* 1968; **i**: 451–3.

(5) Bellman MH, Ross EM, Miller DL. Reye's Syndrome in children under 3 years old. *Arch Dis Childh* 1982; **57**: 259–63.

(6) BPSU third annual report 1988-89 Reye's Syndrome.
(7) Glasgow JFT. Clinical features and prognosis of Reye's Syndrome. *Arch Dis Childh* 1984; **59**: 230–5.
(8) Lyon G, Dodge PR, Adams RD. The acute encephalopathies of obscure origin in infants and children. *Brain* 1961; **84**: 680–708.
(9) Treem WR, Witzleben CA, Ticcoli DA, *et al.* Medium-chain and long-chain acyl CoA dehydrogenase deficiency: clinical pathological and ultrastructural differentiation from Reye's Syndrome. *Hepatology*; **6**: 1270–8.
(10) Lichtenstein PK, Heubi JE, Daugherty CC, *et al.* Grade 1 Reye's Syndrome. A frequent cause of vomiting and liver dysfunction after varicella and upper respiratory tract infection. *N Engl J Med* 1983; **309**: 132–9.
(11) BPSU/CDSC Reye's Syndrome Surveillance Scheme—4th Summary Surveillance Report. Communicable Disease Report 87/33 pages 3–6.
(12) Robinson PH, Glasgow JFT, Moore R. Falling incidence of Reye's Syndrome in Northern Ireland. *Lancet* 1988; **2**: 46.
(13) Glasgow JFT. Unpublished data.
(14) Glasgow JFT, Hicks EM, Jenkins JG, *et al.* Reye's Syndrome. *Br J Hosp Med* 1985; **34**: 42–5.
(15) Wood C, ed. *Reye's syndrome*. London: Royal Society of Medicine Services, Round Table Series No. 8, 1988.
(16) Starko KM, Ray CG, Dominguez LB, *et al.* Reye's syndrome and salicylate use. *Pediatrics* 1980; **66**: 859–64.
(17) Halpin TJ, Holtzhauer FJ, Campbell RJ, *et al.* Reye's Syndrome and medication use. *JAMA* 1982; **248**: 687–91.
(18) Waldman RJ, Hall WN, McGee H, *et al.* Aspirin as a risk factor in Reye's Syndrome. *JAMA* 1982; **247**: 3089–94.
(19) Hall SM. Reye's Syndrome and aspirin: a review. *J Roy Soc Med* 1986; **79**: 596–8.
(20) Hurwitz ES, Barret MJ, Bregman D, *et al.* Public Health Service Study on Reye's Syndrome and medication: Report of the Pilot phase. *N Engl J Med* 1985; **313**: 849–57.
(21) Hurwitz ES, Barret MJ, Bregman D, *et al.* Public Health Service Study on Reye's Syndrome and Medication: Report of the main study. *JAMA* 1987; **257**: 1905–11.
(22) Forsyth BW, Horwitz RA, Acampora D, *et al.* New epidemiologic evidence confirming that bias does not explain the aspirin/Reye's Syndrome association. *JAMA* 1989; **261**: 2517.
(23) Committee on Reye's Syndrome Research. Japanese Ministry of Health and Welfare. Official Report 1983.
(24) Hall SM, Plaster PA, Glasgow JFT, Hancock P. Pre-admission antipyretics in Reye's Syndrome. *Arch Dis Childh* 1988; **63**: 857–66.
(25) Anon. CSM: Reye's Syndrome and Aspirin. *BMJ* 1986; **292**: 1590.
(26) Remington PL, Rowley D, McGee H, *et al.* Decreasing trends in Reye Syndrome and aspirin use in Michigan 1979 to 1984. *Pediatrics* 1986; **77**: 93–8.
(27) Barrett MJ, Hurwitz ES, Shonbergen LB, *et al.* Changing epidemiology of Reye Syndrome in the United States. *Pediatrics* 1986; **77**: 598–602.
(28) Porter JDH, Robinson PH, Glasgow JFT, Hall SM, *et al.* (shortly to be published).

Pathogenic mechanisms of Reye's syndrome

Alex P. Mowat

Department of Child Health, King's College Hospital, London, UK

INTRODUCTION

Paediatricians are indebted to the late Dr Reye. He has made us focus on children with life-threatening or handicapping encephalopathy with hepatic dysfunction. We have learned a great deal in extending his observations. It was he who first brought aspirin into the aetiological argument. The Reye's Syndrome Foundation in Britain is grateful for the help of the aspirin industry with some of the studies which have been conducted in the United Kingdom on Reye's syndrome (RS).

For the purpose of this paper, I will define RS in functional terms, considering the child who has previously been entirely well, in whom all presently known inborn errors of metabolism have been excluded, and who will make a complete recovery from his illness if he avoids the hazards of the encephalopathy.

FUNCTIONAL DEFINITION OF REYE'S SYNDROME

Reye's syndrome is defined as a self-limiting disorder with a defect in all aspects of mitochondrial function and an extremely catabolic state. Endogenous fuel materials are released and are inadequately metabolized, so that toxic metabolites accumulate and further jeopardize the child. The very distorted mitochondria which are pathopneumonic of RS are seen on Day 1, i.e. within 24 h of the onset of the vomiting or encephalopathy. By the fourth day of the illness, the mitochondria are structurally normal and *in vitro* biochemical studies of mitochondrial function suggest that these recover at the same rate.

POSSIBLE CAUSES

What can be doing this? A viral antecedent illness has been suggested, indeed almost every common virus with the exception of measles has been implicated. It is very unusual to recover the virus from the patient, however, and not everyone who gets the viral illness gets RS. There is talk of epidemics of RS in North America, associated with influenza B, perhaps one in 10 000 of those affected by the influenza gets RS and the incidence is much lower even that that with, for example, chicken pox. The virus alone is not responsible for this illness.

Aspirin—towards 2000, edited by G. R. Fryers, 1990; Royal Society of Medicine Services International Congress and Symposium Series No. 168, published by Royal Society of Medicine Services Limited.

Amongst exogenous factors a long list of toxins and drugs has been incriminated and it is interesting that, in the experimental animal, it is possible to show that a virus and some of these agents have additive effects in causing the hepatic mitochondrial abnormality and encephalopathy. Mouse models of RS have included a spontaneous, viral enteritis-associated disorder. Paracetamol with influenza B produced hepatocellular necrosis, but if a mixed-function oxidase-inducer is also given the liver becomes infiltrated with fat. Animal models have also shown insecticides and emulsifiers having no effect on the liver itself but, if given in association with encephalomyocarditis virus, they produced the fatty liver. An association of emulsifiers, aspirin or paracetamol and influenza B, has also caused a Reye's syndrome disorder with a high mortality in mice at two weeks of age but no mortality at five weeks of age, bringing into the experimental field the observation that Reye's syndrome is predominantly a disorder of the young.

There is also considerable evidence that chemical agents interact with viruses to potentiate their deleterious effects and this works both ways. Could something like this be happening in Reye's syndrome? If so, how could it occur? There are many examples we could quote of the interaction between viruses and disruption of differentiated cell function, for example, in lymphocytes the measles virus has a well-demonstrated effect of causing loss of natural killer cell activity. Both measles and influenza virus decrease immunoglobulin synthesis on differentiated cells. There are many well-documented abnormalities of this type, affecting the immune system particularly, following viral infection.

Indeed, in Reye's syndrome we do have some immunological abnormalities such as low complement levels, reduced fibronectin concentrations and reduced interferon production. Fibronectin's main function is usually considered to be as a supportive, structural, non-functioning protein but it is now known that there are specific fibronectin receptors on the hepatocyte through which the fibronectin influences intrahepatic metabolism. Thus, we have a direct link between the immune system and the hepatocyte. In the time available it is not possible to consider all of the possible interactions which may occur. Exogenous factors may influence the functioning of the immune system e.g. the effects of aspirin on some of the lymphokines, the chemicals that interconnect the whole immune process. This may occur at any stage from the antigen-presenting cell through to the critical T-helper cell, the controlling cell for all cellular immune responses, to the effector cells, e.g. the killer cells or the antigen-producing B-cells.

Why are the mitochondria selected for attack, when all the other subcellular particles appear normal? We have no answer to this, but it is as well to remember that the mitochondria do share a lot of features with bacteria, and perhaps we are getting a direct viral effect, something like a phage virus effect, on mitochondria.

The other possibility, however, is that there is interference with mitochondrial function, secondary to an effect on another part of the hepatocyte. One possibility is an effect on the protein membrane. This is derived from proteins synthesized in the cell cytoplasm, which are transported into the mitochondria where they are modified by proteases before being incorporated into the structure of the mitochondrial wall. This wall appears to be absolutely essential for all mitochondrial functions.

THE CATABOLIC STATE

The other major pathogenic factor in RS is the severe catabolic state. At present, we do not have an explanation for this. Whether it is some response to the virus which has initiated the condition we really do not know, but there seems little doubt that the onset of vomiting, which is a characteristic feature of RS, and the fasting that goes with it, must have a tremendous effect on the load that the mitochondria carries. As fasting continues in a young child, the carbohydrate reserves are rapidly used up and more and more fat is mobilized to provide metabolic needs. Remembering the range of metabolic processes occurring in fatty acids in the mitochondria, and that all of these are disturbed in RS, one could very easily see the patient becoming overloaded with metabolites, e.g. dicarboxylic acids, some of which are toxic.

THE ENCEPHALOPATHY

We do not know what causes the encephalopathy. There are a few observations suggesting that the mitochondrial abnormality, seen clearly in the liver, also occurs in the brain. We know that fatty acids can affect particularly the endothelial cells of the vessels in the brain; we do know that there is defective oxidative phosphorylation of glucose transport in the brain in RS but whether that is secondary to the hepatic lesion or not we do not know. Ammonia and fatty acids accumulate and there is hypoglycaemia; all three of these can produce encephalopathy in experimental animals. It is perhaps an interaction of all of these, but we really do not know.

SUMMARY

At present we do not know very much about the pathogenesis of RS. We do know that it is a self-limiting disorder of mitochondrial function and structure, associated with an extreme catabolic rate. I have speculated on some of the factors that might be involved in causing this, and at present our hypothesis is that the cause may be a virus plus an exogenous agent or agents interacting with some host factor which seems to be age-related; there may be dietary components or undiagnosed genetic factors, all of them leading to a mitochondrial membrane defect to produce this challenging syndrome.

DISCUSSION

Dr Smith: It is difficult to understand a genetic or inborn error of metabolism in cases where there is such sharp age-related symptomatology. You are postulating really an inborn error of metabolism which will reverse and become normal in a child of nine months in Britain or 12 years in the USA. How do you explain that?

Dr Mowat: Perhaps the next speaker will address this, but one thing we have learned in recent years concerns, for example, the urea cycle defects which were initially described in newborn infants as a devastating illness. Somewhat similar disorders and the same biochemical abnormality sometimes present in late teens and early 20s, so that there is a periodicity to some of these metabolic disorders which I certainly do not understand. However, if you stress these patients appropriately, you can demonstrate the biochemical abnormality and, of course, with the advent of genetic markers for metabolic abnormalities we expect to document even more of them. Furthermore, RS has now been described in adults.

Dr Glasgow: One of the difficulties that we have, I think, is the question that has just been put. How does one begin to tackle this problem: how can we take our understanding further in this area? Do you think that the patients who have already suffered Reye's syndrome and are, as it were, still available for investigation, hold the key to our understanding? The patients we are seeing at the moment with Reye's syndrome, I understand, are much less convincing cases than those we were seeing three or four years ago. I wonder where we should be making our effort in advancing our understanding?

Dr Mowat: One of the difficulties in answering this question is that it is much less than the 25% you showed as having liver biopsies who have actually had electron microscopy done on the liver, so we really do not know how big the problem of Reye's syndrome as I have defined it might be. We have seen over the years a progressive recognition of more and more metabolic abnormalities that are separated from idiopathic Reye's syndrome. I am sure we must cooperate more closely with those who are studying inborn errors of metabolism as their prime pursuit.

Dr Lockhart: You mentioned that you were able to see the change in the mitochondria within 24 h of the onset of the symptoms. Is there any evidence at all about how early you can see the mitochondrial changes; can you see them in the prodromal period?

Dr Mowat: I do not have any answer to that question. However, it is very interesting that in the study characterizing RS Grade I, some of the patients who were only a little drowsy and showed no other features of encephalopathy, had similar electron microscopic abnormalities.

REFERENCE

(1) Heubi JE, Daugherty CC, Partin JS, Partin JC, Schubert WK. Grade one Reye's Syndrome—outcome and predictors of progression to deeper coma grades. *N Engl J Med* 1988; **331**: 1539–42.

The relationship of inborn errors of metabolism to Reye's and Reye-like syndromes

Priscille Divry

Unite d'Etude des Maladies Metaboliques, Hôpital Debrousse, Lyon, France

INTRODUCTION

We are a large team involved in all inborn errors of metabolism, covering the south of France and, for some very rare conditions, a much wider area. We undertake enzymatic and cell culture studies, and I am involved in amino-acid metabolism and organic acid metabolism. In the last six years we have diagnosed nearly 100 patients with organic acidurias and some of these diseases mimic the presentation of Reye's syndrome.

A Reye-like syndrome presentation has been reported in a great number of inborn errors of metabolism, especially in metabolism located inside the mitochondria, including urea cycle defects, branched chain amino-acid metabolism and related organic acidurias, and mitochondrial fatty acid β-oxidation (Table 1).

UREA CYCLE DEFECTS

Most of the inborn errors located on urea cycle metabolism classically have a neonatal presentation, but it must be kept in mind that a late-onset form can occur in all of them, in ornithine transcarbamylase (OTC) deficiency, in carbamylphosphate synthesis deficiency, in citrullinaemia, and even in argininosuccinic aciduria, which has been reported as a Reye-like syndrome in an 11-years-old child (1).

ORNITHINE TRANSCARBAMYLASE DEFICIENCY

OTC deficiency is probably the most important in this respect. A Reye-like syndrome has been described in late-onset form in boys and OTC heterozygote carriers in girls (2,3). We have experienced this with four OTC patients, two boys and two girls, who presented in inaugural coma. One of the girls, 12 years old, had Reye's syndrome initiated by valproate therapy. She recovered promptly but, afterwards the history of protein aversion and poor weight gain during infancy drew the attention of the paediatrician. An oral load test with protein was performed and demonstrated the excretion of orotic acid in urine and a partial OTC deficiency was then confirmed.

Aspirin—towards 2000, edited by G. R. Fryers, 1990; Royal Society of Medicine Services International Congress and Symposium Series No. 168, published by Royal Society of Medicine Services Limited.

Table 1 *Metabolic disorders with Reye-like syndrome presentation*

1. **Ureagenesis**
   Partial OTC deficiency
   Partial CPS deficiency
   Argininosuccinate synthetase deficiency
   Citrullinaemia
   Lysinuric protein intolerance (LPI)
   Hyperammonaemia, Hyperornithinaemia and Homocitrullinuria (HHH)

2. **Branched chain amino acid metabolism**
   Propionic acidaemia
   Methylmalonic acidaemia
   Isovaleric acidaemia
   3-hydroxy-3-methylglutaric aciduria
   3-methylcrotonyl CoA carboxylase deficiency
   Holocarboxylase synthetase deficiency
   Biotinidase deficiency

3. **Fatty oxidation**
   Various acyl CoA dehydrogenase deficiencies
      Medium chain MCAD
      Long chain LCAD
      Multiple MAD
      Long chain 3-OH acyl CoA DH
   Primary carnitine deficiency
   Hepatic carnitine palmityl transferase deficiency

4. **Miscellaneous**
   Fructose 1.6 diphosphate
   Hereditary fructose intolerance
   Glutaric acidaemia type I
   Hereditary adrenocortical unresponsiveness to ACTH

The same history of the diagnosis of an inborn error after valproate induction of a Reye's syndrome has recently been reported in France in an adult man of 22 years who attempted suicide with valproate. He had a classic Reye's syndrome and after recovery, a 50% activity of carbamylphosphate synthesis was found in his liver biopsy (4).

BRANCHED CHAIN AMINO ACID INBORN ERRORS

The second group of inborn errors which can mimic Reye's syndrome involves branched chain amino acid metabolism. Elevation of short chain fatty acid in the plasma of Reye's syndrome patients was described about 14 years ago (5). At the same time, as more cases of propionic and methylmalonic acidaemia were described, it became obvious that severe hyperammonaemia was a constant finding in these disorders. In fact, in the literature not many cases have been reported associated with Reye's syndrome presentation, except for 3-hydroxy-3-methylglutaric aciduria, of which five cases have been reported (6–9) and isolated 3 methylcrotonyl CoA carboxylase (10). However, it is quite clear that the clinical presentation in late-onset patients can mimic Reye's syndrome. There is encephalopathy after vomiting and fever, hypoglycaemia, hyperammonaemia, and acidosis with or without ketosis.

In our own experience, of 21 cases of propionic acidaemia, four had an inaugural coma when aged 3–4 years, and two were referred to our hospital with the diagnosis of Reye's syndrome. In methylmalonic acidaemia, out of 20 patients six had a late-onset, four with an inaugural coma at 16 months, 18 months, three years and four years respectively. Isovaleric acidaemia can also mimic Reye's syndrome: we have now had 11 patients, three with late onset. We have also the opportunity to diagnose an holocarboxylase synthetase deficiency with a late onset decompensation in a Reye-like coma. Other disorders have been listed, such as biotinidase deficiency, of which I have no experience. Ketothiolase deficiency is also listed in a publication (11) about Reye's syndrome and metabolic disorders but, in my opinion, the clinical presentation is very different. There is a huge ketoacidosis, glycaemia is normal or elevated, ammonia is normal or very low, and the differential diagnosis is not Reye's syndrome but diabetic coma or aspirin poisoning.

An explanation of the hyperammonaemia in those disorders of organic acidaemia was demonstrated in 1979 (12). The propionyl coenzyme A (CoA) accumulated in the mitochondria in propionic acidaemia has a competitive inhibitor to the synthesis of n-acetyl glutamase (NAGA) which is an effector of the first enzyme of the urea cycle. Other acyl CoAs have been shown to be inhibitors, but propionyl CoA is the strongest one. The same inhibition mechanism applies to valproyl CoA, the metabolite of valproate. It is very important to remember that acetyl CoA will be depleted in all this group of disorders leading to a low rate of n-acetyl glutamate synthesis. Moreover, the lack of acetyl CoA inside the mitochondria will depress the pyruvate carboxylase, thus limiting the aspartate concentration and also the arginine concentration and so depressing all the urea cycle.

DISORDERS OF CARBOHYDRATE METABOLISM

Some disorders of carbohydrate metabolism can mimic Reye's syndrome, especially fructose 1,6-diphosphatase deficiency with acute presentation: hypoglycaemias, hepatomegaly, liver dysfunction and fatty liver. It also has been reported in one case of fructose intolerance (13).

MISCELLANEOUS

Another disorder, glutaric acidaemia Type I is quite different. It is a progressive neurological disease with psychomotor regression and ataxia, but some acute episodes of metabolic dysfunction have been reported and we have diagnosed glutaric acidaemia Type I six months after death, in a frozen urine sample from a Reye-like patient. It was a four-years old girl found comatose in her bed in the morning, who died some hours afterwards in hospital (14).

The last disease in this group is also quite different: Hereditary adrenocortical unresponsiveness to adrenocorticotrophic hormone (ACTH). The patient was a four-years-old boy from consanguinous parents who developed progressive coma with hyperammonaemia and hypoglycaemia. Diagnosis was made after death by the pathologist who discovered very abnormal adrenal glands. In 1986 two other cases, two brothers, were reported by pathologists from University Hospital of Madison USA (15) supporting the hypothesis of an X-linked mode of inheritance.

All the inborn errors mentioned so far can mimic Reye's syndrome, they are Reye-like syndromes, they sometimes have slightly different clinical course than Reye's syndrome. Except for the latter they are very easy to diagnose on urinary organic acid profile and/or amino acids analysis.

FATTY OXIDATION DEFECTS

Fatty oxidation defects are much more important and more closely related to Reye's syndrome. They were first identified in 1976 (16) so they are rather a new group of diseases. They were first called dicarboxylic acidurias because of the presence of these metabolites in urine. Medium-chain acyl CoA dehydrogenase deficiency (MCAD) was the first deficiency to be described and is the most frequent, there are now more than 100 cases in the literature, and probably there are many more because nobody any longer publishes them. MCAD has been very

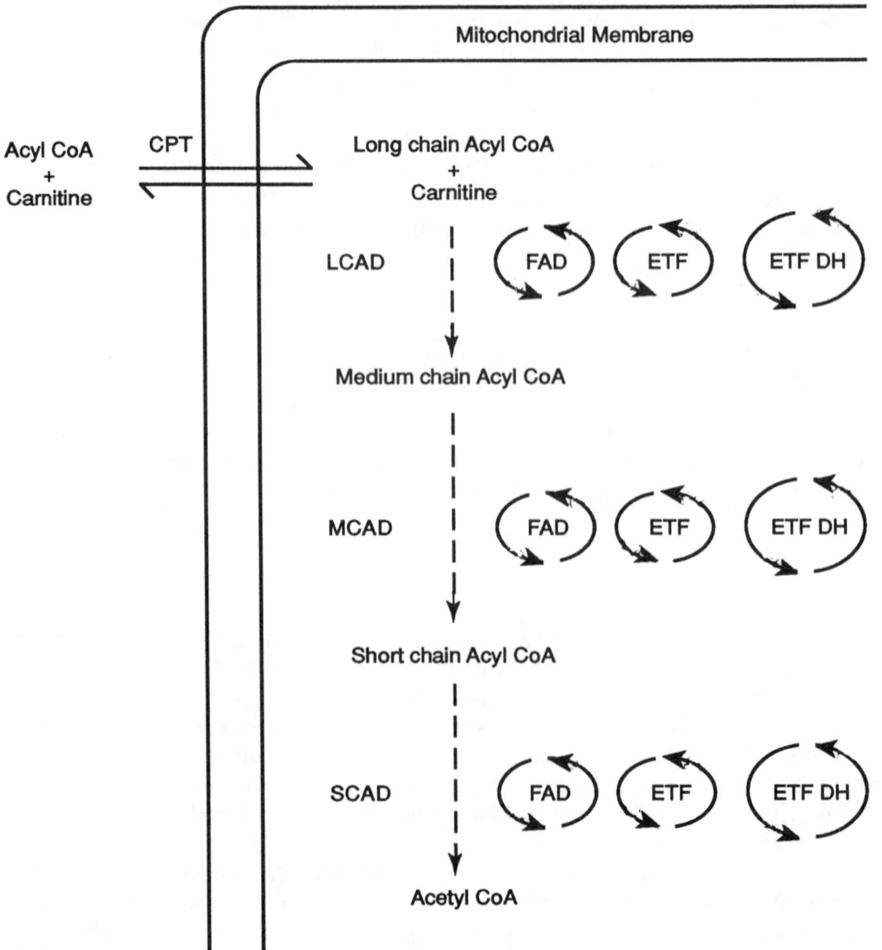

Figure 1 *Inborn defects of mitochondrial β-oxidation: simplified scheme of their localization.*

often described in siblings of patients who die of Reye's syndrome or of sudden infant death. About 20–25 cases are reported as Reye's syndrome in the literature (17–21). The other inborn errors, long-chain acyl CoA dehydrogenase deficiency (LCAD) and multiple acyl CoA dehydrogenase deficiency (MAD), hepatic carnitine palmityltransferase (CPT) deficiency and primary carnitine deficiency, are much more difficult to diagnose; there are only a few cases reported but they also can have a presentation of Reye's syndrome.

Mitochondrial β-oxidation pathway is illustrated in Fig. 1. At least seven different inborn errors have been demonstrated. They have been reviewed recently (22). Dysfunction of this metabolism can involve insufficient carnitine supply to the cell, or deficiency of the carnitine palmityltransferase (CPT) the enzyme which makes the fatty acyl CoA enter the mitochondria. Then takes place the β-oxidation which degrades C^{16} fatty acids to C^2 (acetyl CoA). In this process are involved three different dehydrogenases: a long chain (LCAD), a medium chain (MCAD), a short chain (SCAD). The transport of electrons to the respiratory chain is common to all the dehydrogenases and involves: an electron transfer flavoprotein (ETF) and ETF dehydrogenase (ETFDH). The lack of one of these transporters is responsible for the multiple acyl CoA dehydrogenase deficiency (MAD).

The typical block of β-oxidation, deficiency of the MCAD, especially at the octanoyl CoA level (Fig. 2), causes microsomal β-oxidation giving dicarboxylic acids that are then β-oxidized by the peroxisome and octanoyl carnitine, hexanoyl glycine and suberyl glycine are found in the urine. These metabolites are very specific to MCAD deficiency. Elevated values of acyl carnitines in urine is a common feature of all these diseases. The separation and identification of the specific acyl carnitines (for example: octanoyl carnitine, isovaleryl carnitine) is a very diagnostically useful technique. Carnitine serves to excrete from the mitochondria the toxic acyl CoA accumulated. L Carnitine therapy is used in many organic acidurias and has been proposed in Reye's syndrome (23).

All the features present in these fatty oxidation defects have been also found in Reye's syndrome. That is, free fatty acid elevation in plasma, dicarboxylic aciduria, dicarboxylic acid carnitines (24) and elevation of medium and short chain fatty acyl CoA esters in the liver (25).

A recent study from the USA (26) illustrates the similarities between β-oxidation defects and Reye's syndrome. It included 12 patients with MCAD and three with LCAD deficiency: six of them have been referred with a Reye's syndrome diagnosis. According to the author, all (100%) had lethargy, hypoglycaemia, hyperammonaemia and transaminase elevation, so that if they were not real Reye's syndrome they were a Reye-like syndrome.

This study emphasizes the need for metabolic investigation to diagnose these inborn errors of oxidation, urinary organic acid profile with gas chromatography-mass spectrometry (GC-MS) can easily diagnose MCAD because of the specific hexanoyl, suberyl and phenylpropionyl glycine, but the urine must be taken as soon as possible as this specific profile disappears rapidly after glucose therapy. The other disorders are more difficult to diagnose, the dicarboxylic acid profile is not specific and enzymatic study in fibroblasts is actually the only way to diagnose these defects.

In conclusion, the importance of metabolic investigations in the Reye's syndrome is emphasized in a recent paper by Rowe in December 1988 (9). They described four Reye's syndrome patients referred for monitoring, all of whom were in fact suffering from metabolic disease. There was one partial OTC deficiency in a 12-year-old girl, MCAD deficiency in a two-year-old, a 3-hydroxy-3-methyl-glutaric aciduria in a four-months-old girl and another OTC deficiency in a nine-months-old boy.

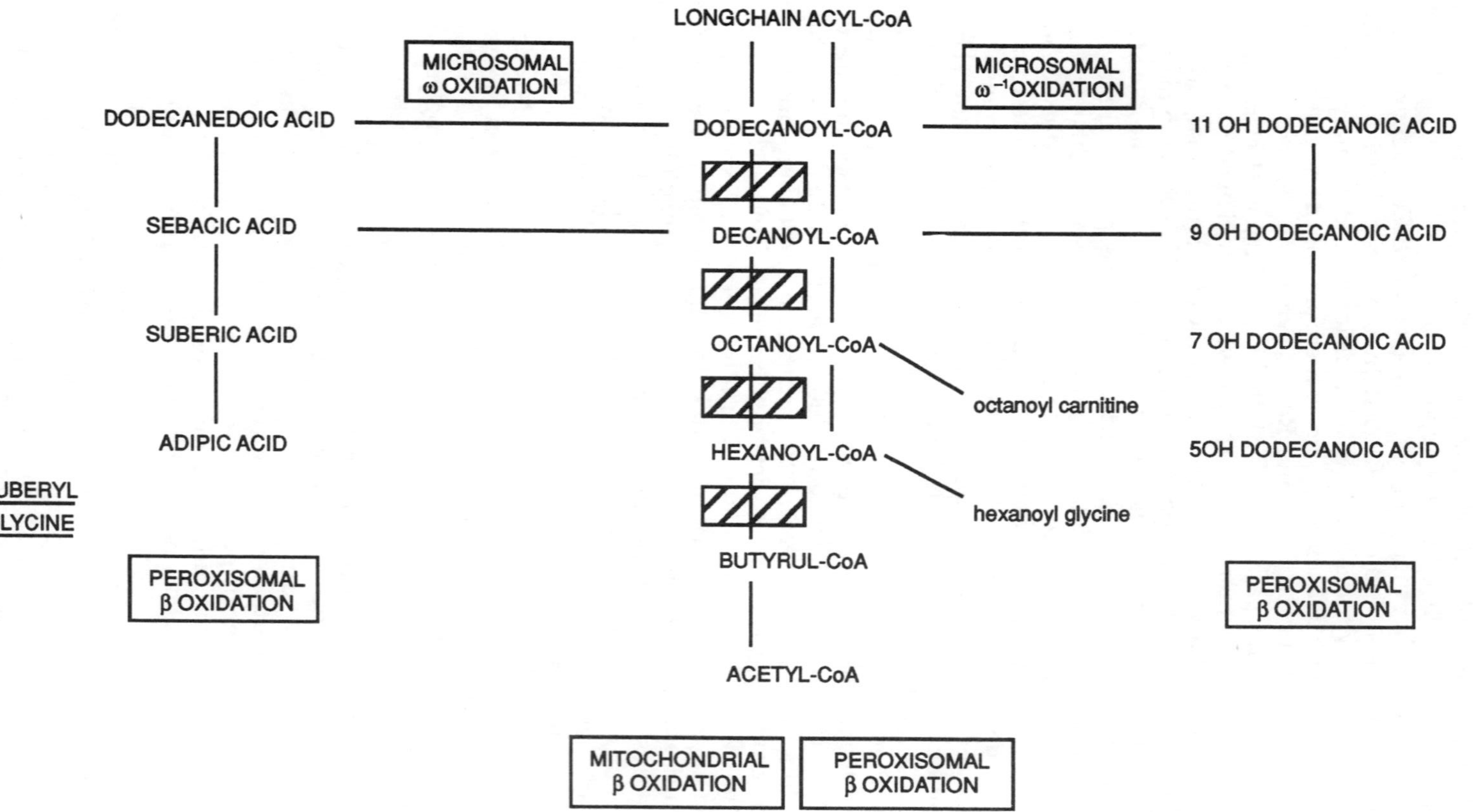

Figure 2 *MCAD deficiency: simplified metabolic scheme proposed for the alternative metabolic processes (according to Gregersen, 1984). In fact, mitochondrial and peroxisomal β-oxidation act on acyl-CoA, while microsomal ω— and ω—1-oxidation act on free fatty acids. The defective steps in the normal pathway of fatty acid β-oxidation are marked with hatched squares. Metabolites excreted in urine are underlined (from Vianey-Liaud* et al. *1987).*

PERSONAL EXPERIENCE

In France there is no register for Reye's syndrome, so there are no statistics about Reye's syndrome and inborn errors of metabolism, even in my own hospital. The reason is simple: in our hospital all the patients have a metabolic investigation with at least plasma amino acids and urinary organic acid profile. The diagnosis will be given in 6–12 h so these patients, if the diagnosis is positive, will directly be registered as inborn errors and will not appear as Reye's syndrome.

The protocol for metabolic investigation in our hospital has been operating since 1984 (Table 2). We provide the intensive care unit with a box containing all the collection tubes and sampling material ready to use, with clear instructions. This is to help the staff who have a thousand things to do in those dramatic situations. Among those analyses the more important are organic acid in urine, amino acid in plasma, and perhaps orotic acid in urine. Free fatty acid, lactate and pyruvate is of interest for the intermediary metabolism as a help to diagnosis, and the medium chain fatty acids are useful for MCAD deficiency. In most cases a skin biopsy is taken for fibroblast culture and if the patient dies we try to have liver and muscle biopsies, not only for pathology but also for enzyme studies.

An example of a Reye-like case was a girl who was hospitalized when she was three years of age after a one-month history of bronchitis and upper respiratory tract infection and a 24 h history of vomiting. She arrived in coma with dehydration, ketoacidosis, hyperammonaemia, normal transaminases, glycaemia was not very low. On the urinary organic acid profile we found: methyl citrate, tiglyl glycine, propionyl glycine, we had also aspirin metabolites and there was a typical propionic acidaemia. In fact this child had received aspirin before and it is not aspirin that leads to the Reye's syndrome, but the history of all this disease with vomiting, leading to proteolysis, and a catabolic state. Also, she had been fasting and that is a precipitating factor.

Another child was also four years old when she arrived at our hospital in coma and dehydrated, with no previous history. She had decreased coagulation factor, and she was discharged after rehydration. She came back one month later with another coma after a history of vomiting. She had ketoacidosis, hyperammonaemia, normal transaminases, slight hypoglycaemia, but a strong odour of sweaty feet and this was an isovaleric acidaemia.

A further case was rather more complicated. A nine months' old girl was hospitalized in Strasbourg (Pr Juif-Dr Burstcher), after three days of diarrhoea and hypotonia and dehydration she was in coma with ketoacidosis, a very strong acidosis, a very severe hypoglycaemia, hyperammonaemia, and normal transaminases. She was treated by alkalination, glucose and intravenous carnitine. This gave some clinical improvement but did not correct the acidosis.

Table 2 *Reye's syndrome. Protocol of investigation for diagnosis of inborn errors*

Plasma	Urines
● Amino acids	● Organic acids
● Medium chain fatty acids (C8, C10, C10 : 1)	● Orotic acid
● NEFA	● Amino acids
● Lactate, pyruvate	● Reducing sugars
● 3-OH butyrate, acetoacetate	● Carnitine
● Carnitine	
SKIN BIOPSY: room temperature (fibroblast culture)	
LIVER, MUSCLE (HEART, . . .) BIOPSY: −80°C (enzyme studies)	

Urinary organic acids referred to us showed huge peaks of lactic acid, 3-hydroxy-isovaleric acid and 3-methylcrotonyl-glycine, giving a strong suspicion of multi-carboxylase deficiency. A blood sample was taken for enzyme studies and sent to Basel to R. Baumgartner, and it was found to be a holocarboxylase synthetase deficiency. It is very important to diagnose this kind of disorder because the children can be resuscitated by biotin therapy in a few hours.

Our experience with medium-chain acyl CoA dehydrogenase is similar to others. We have seen six patients in five families and in these families there were two previous deaths (sudden infant deaths), two Reye's syndromes, one Near-Miss presentation, one acute hypoglycaemic coma, one history of recurrent hypoglycaemias since birth, and one is an asymptomatic sibling of this patient. Those are fairly easy to diagnose with organic acid profiles in urine, but now we must consider other defects of β-oxidation which are much more difficult to diagnose. We had one very curious story: a family history of myocardiopathy with lipid storage myopathy and low carnitine values, following which the second brother arrived in our hospital with a Reye's syndrome at eight months and we found little of importance in the urine. Carnitine was very low in plasma, and it was the enzymatic study in fibroblasts that gave the clue: a defective oxidation of palmitate (50% of controls) corrected by addition of L Carnitine *in vitro*. The defect, first described last year by the Philadelphia Group (27) is a 'primary carnitine deficiency', characterized by a decreased uptake of carnitine by the cells.

Another case, also a Reye's syndrome at eight months from which he recovered, had a very low carnitine value in plasma at 11 months, indicating a strong suspicion of β-oxidation defect. At 16 months he was referred to the hospital because of fever. When arriving he had hepatomegaly, but the glycaemia was normal, and he was found dead during the night, five hours later, with a Dextrostix=zero. The dicarboxylic aciduria was impressive and this child also had a decrease of palmitate oxidation in fibroblasts. It is probably a 3-hydroxy long-chain acyl CoA dehydrogenase deficiency, but that is not yet confirmed as only two or three laboratories in the world are able to perform this assay.

Our experience of the diagnosis of many different inborn errors among children referred for Reye or Reye-like presentation does not imply that we get a diagnosis for all the Reye patients. In the last seven years we have seen about 11 cases (five in our hospital, six from other hospitals) without any diagnosis, despite accurate analysis of urinary organic acids and plasma amino acids. But for most of them we do not have skin biopsies and we were not able to go further with sophisticated enzyme studies.

Recurrent Reye's syndrome is another problem. We have been studying three patients with recurrent Reye's syndrome without diagnosis despite extensive investigations. One of these patients is specially puzzling. He is from probably consanguineous parents and developed the first Reye's syndrome when he was five years old. He had a second Reye's syndrome some time later, from which he died. The first urine we obtained was one day after the first episode and there was nothing except aspirin and a huge peak I could not identify. The second urine obtained during the second episode was the same: aspirin, but the huge peak was identified as thenoyl glycine. Thenoyl glycine is from thenoic acid, a constituent of a drug called 'Trophirès', widely used in France for children with fever and respiratory tract infection. Thenoyl glycine is a normal metabolite, however it raises the question of metabolization via CoA ester and glycine conjunction inside the mitochondria.

CONCLUSION

Metabolic investigation should be done in all patients and not only in special patients with recurrent Reye's syndrome, as has previously been suggested. It should include at least a plasma sample, a urine sample taken before therapy or soon after. If no urine is available cerebrospinal fluid can be useful. If there is rapid death, of course it should be taken *post mortem* as should skin biopsy for fibroblast culture and liver for enzyme study.

The results should be available rapidly because this will lead to specific therapy and/or diet. Moreover, even a post mortem analysis and diagnosis is important for genetic counselling and, in some cases, possibility of therapy at birth or of antenatal diagnosis.

It must be kept in mind, that: 'Although each of these inborn errors of metabolism are rare, they are as a group at least as common as Reye syndrome' (11).

REFERENCES

(1) Guertin SR, Levinsohn MW, Dahms BB. Small droplet steatosis and intracranial hypertension in arginino-succinic lyase deficiency. *J Pediatr* 1983; **102**: 736–40.

(2) Krieger I, Snodgrass PJ, Roskamo J. Atypical clinical course of ornithine transcarbamylase deficiency due to a new mutant (comparison with Reye's disease). *J Clin Endocrinol Metab* 1979; **48**: 388–92.

(3) Yokoi T, Honke K, Funabashi T, *et al.* Partial ornithine transcarbamylase deficiency simulating Reye syndrome. *J Pediatr* 1981; **99**: 929–31.

(4) Bourrier P, Varache N, Alquier P, *et al.* Oedeme cerebral avec hyperammoniamie au cours d'une intoxication par le Valpromide. Revelation, chez un adulte d'un deficit partiel en carbamylphosphate synthetase de type I. *Presse Medicale* 1988; **17**(No. 39): 2063–6.

(5) Trauner DA, Nyhan WL, Sweetman L. Short chain organic acidemia and Reye's syndrome. *Neurology* 1975; **25**: 296–8.

(6) Robinson PH, Oei J, Sherwood WG, Slyper AH, Heininger J, Mamer OA. Hydroxymethylglutaryl CoA lyase deficiency features resembling Reye syndrome. *Neurology* 1980; **30**: 714–8.

(7) Leonard JV, Seakins JWT, Griffin NK. Beta hydroxy beta methylglutaricaciduria presenting as Reye's syndrome (Letter). *Lancet* 1979; **i**: 680.

(8) Leonard JV, Seakins JWT, Griffin NK, Marshall WC. Beta-hydroxy-beta methylglutaricaciduria. Reye's syndrome and Echovirus II (Letter). *Lancet* 1979; **i**: 1147.

(9) Rowe PC, Valle D, Brusilow SW. Inborn errors of metabolism in children referred with Reye's syndrome. A changing pattern. *JAMA* 1988; **260**: 3167–70.

(10) Kobori JA, Johnston K, Sweetman L, *et al.* Isolated 3-methylcrotonyl CoA carboxylase deficiency presenting as a Reye's-like syndrome. *Ped Res* 1989; no. 2: 836 [abstract].

(11) Greene CL, Blitzer MG, Shapira E. Inborn errors of metabolism and Reye Syndrome: differential diagnosis. *J Pediatr* 1988; **113**: 156–9.

(12) Coude FX, Sweetman L, Nyhan WL. Inhibition by propionyl-coenzyme A of N-acetylglutamate synthetase in rat liver mitochondria. *J Clin Invest* 1979; **64**: 1544–51.

(13) Gitzelmann R, Steinmann B, Van Den Berghe G. Hereditary fructose intolerance. In: Stanbury JB, ed. *The metabolic basis of inherited disease,* 5th Ed. New York: McGraw-Hill, 1983.

(14) Floret D, Divry P, Dingeon N, Monnet P. Acidurie glutarique: une nouvelle observation. *Arch Franc Pediat* 1979; **36**: 462–70.

(15) Sunita-Chandra, Gilbert EF. Hereditary adrenocortical unresponsiveness to adrenocorticotropic hormone. *Pediatric Pathology Symposium* Dallas, Oct. 1986. [Abstract].

(16) Gregersen N, Lauritzen R, Rasmussen K. Suberyl glycine excretion in the urine from a patient with dicarboxylic aciduria. *Clin Chim Acta* 1976; **70**: 417–25.
(17) Del Valle JA, Garcia MJ, Merinero B, *et al.* A new patient with dicarboxylic aciduria suggestive of medium chain acyl CoA dehydrogenase deficiency presenting as Reye's syndrome. *J Inher Metab Dis* 1984; **7**: 62–4.
(18) Stanley CA, Coates PM. Inherited defects of fatty acid oxidation which resemble Reye's syndrome. *J Natl Reye's Syndrome Foundation* 1985; **5**: 190–200.
(19) Bougneres PF, Rocchiccioli F, Kolvraa S, *et al.* Medium-chain acyl-CoA dehydrogenase deficiency in two siblings with a Reye-like syndrome. *J Pediatr* 1985; **106**: 918–21.
(20) Roe CR, Millington DS, Maltby DA, *et al.* Recognition of medium chain acyl CoA dehydrogenase deficiency in asymptomatic siblings of children dying of sudden infant death or Reye-like syndromes. *J Pediatr* 1986; **108**: 13–18.
(21) Taubmann B, Hale DE, Kelly RI. Familial Reye-like syndrome: a presentation of medium-chain acyl-Coenzyme A dehydrogenase deficiency. *Pediatrics* 1987; **79**: 382–5.
(22) Vianey-Liaud C, Divry P, Gregersen N, Mathieu M. The inborn errors of mitochondrial fatty acid oxidation. *J Inher Metab Dis* 1987; **10**(suppl 1): 159–98.
(23) Stumpf DA, Parker WDJ, Angelini C. Carnitine deficiency, organic acidaemias and Reye's syndrome. *Neurology* 1985; **35**: 1041–5.
(24) Tracey BM, Cheng KN, Rosankiewicz J, Stacey JE, Chalmers RA. Urinary C6–C12 dicarboxylic acylcarnitines in Reye's syndrome. *Clin Chim Acta* 1988; **175**: 79–88.
(25) Corkey BE, Hale DA, Glennon MC, *et al.* Relationship between unusual hepatic Acyl Coenzyme A profiles and the pathogenesis of Reye Syndrome. *J Clin Invest* 1988; **82**: 782–8.
(26) Treem WR, Witzleben CA, Piccoli DA, *et al.* Medium chain and long chain Acyl CoA dehydrogenase deficiency: clinical, pathologic and ultrastructural differentiation from Reye's syndrome. *Hepatology* 1986; **6**: 1270–8.
(27) Treem WR, Stanley CA, Finegold DN, Hale DE, Coates PM. Primary carnitine deficiency due to a failure of carnitine transport in kidney muscle and fibroblasts. *N Engl J Med* 1988; **319**: 1331–6.

DISCUSSION

Dr Lockhart: It appears that you can diagnose just about every child with Reye-like syndrome: is that correct?

Dr Divry: No, not every child. We have some children undiagnosed even after GC-MS (Gas Chromatography-Mass Spectrometry) analysis of urine. We have 12–13 Reye-like syndrome patients without any diagnosis.

Dr Lockhart: It appears that Reye's syndrome occurs in certain areas: Dr Glasgow mentioned that Northern Ireland has a higher incidence than the rest of the UK, for instance. It appears also in the USA that the incidence is greater in the mid-West than it is in other areas. Could this be due to hereditary factors that exist in these populations? Some countries say they do not even see it.

Dr Divry: I cannot answer this question.

Dr Glasgow: Why is there a geographical selectivity for Reye's syndrome in certain areas of the USA, whereas in other countries they scarcely see the condition at all, for example France.

Dr Divry: In France it is known that there are not many Reye's syndrome cases. I have discussed this with Professor Saudubray from Paris, from where most

French cases come. In his opinion there should be only 10–20 a year in France, but perhaps it is true that the diagnostic criteria are not exactly the same in our hospitals. It is not called Reye's syndrome if patients do not have hepatic microvesicular steatosis. If there is no liver biopsy physicians will not say it is Reye's syndrome, so maybe that is one of the differences. In my opinion, there may also be a difference because it depends on the means of investigation available to look for inborn errors. I do not know whether there is a geographical difference.

Dr Mowat: In which of these metabolic disorders would you expect aspirin to have an added deleterious effect on metabolism in acute exacerbation? Also, in Reye's syndrome disorders that you did not diagnose, had you done electron microscopy of the liver in the acute phase?

Dr Divry: To the second question, I am not sure that we had in those undiagnosed patients a clear hepatology study. Also, it is clear from these patients that for most of them we do not have fibroblasts so we cannot go further in our fibroblast studies. They had nothing on screening urinary organic acid and amino acids. On the first question, I do not know about the effect of aspirin. I have seen about 4000 urines from ill children for GC-MS analysis. Many of them have had aspirin metabolites in them. I know that in these kinds of inborn errors, all drugs that are metabolized with acyl CoA derivatives can be toxic—valproate, thenoic acid, benzoic acid. Benzoic acid has been used widely for urea cycle disease and it may be very toxic for organic acidaemia, because the benzoate will trap acyl CoA from the mitochondria. But for aspirin I do not know. Aspirin metabolism probably involves acyl CoA because you have the salicyluric metabolite, so you have a glycine conjugate and you should pass by an acyl CoA metabolite.

Dr de Gaetano: What evidence exists that aspirin rather than salicylates or other metabolites is involved in Reye's syndrome, and is there any evidence that giving prostaglandins, for instance PGE_1 or PGE_2 or prostacyclin, gives any clinical improvement in these patients?

Dr Divry: I have no idea about prostaglandins.

Dr Glasgow: As far as I know there is no such evidence. Most of the work has been related to aspirin itself rather than salicylates and there are very few data in any of the epidemiological studies on the use of non-aspirin salicylates, for example the teething gels and so on. As far as I know there are no data on prostaglandins.

Unidentified: Do children with such errors of metabolism reach adult age and, if so, is their condition an extra risk factor if they take aspirin in maturity?

Dr Divry: Some of them can reach maturity. There are so many inborn errors that I cannot answer the general question, because some, like the neonatal form of propionic acidaemia, nearly all die when they are 1–2 years old even when monitored, but when they develop the late-onset form they can reach maturity. We have a propionic acidaemia patient who is now 22 years old. I think the major problem for these people is not aspirin but fasting, vomiting and catabolic states, because the proteolysis and the catabolic state cause the amino acids to be catabolized and then there is accumulation of abnormal metabolites. However, you have adult patients with urea cycle defects, partially defective, and with β-oxidation defects. The mean age of MCAD deficiency is 1–2 years. That means that these children are perfect for a long time unless they are obliged to use their lipid store for fuel. They are quite perfect until they have to fast for any reason, when they deplete their glucose and their glycogen and shift their fuel to fatty acid oxidation. Then within six hours they will develop a strong hypoglycaemic coma and Reye-like syndrome, or a sudden infant death.

Dr Glasgow: As far as we understand it at present, fasting and catabolism seem to be worse than aspirin.

Dr Fryers: When you give aspirin, most of it is in the peripheral circulation as sodium salicylate rather than as aspirin, and there are two anomalies about the aspirin association data in this regard. One major one is that we do not really have any evidence of a dose-response relationship. Also, in considering whether aspirin was used or not, normally a very wide span of time has been chosen, like 10 days. If it was given at all, even just once in the 10 days, it is regarded as having been given, but there is no mechanism that we know of by which aspirin would act after 10 days: even the platelet mechanism which is not suggested in this regard. So the development of Reye's syndrome can often occur well after the aspirin was given and the whole process still seems to be shrouded in mystery.

Dr Glasgow: It is a very complex area, from the diagnostic criteria which are woolly, to the involvement of exogenous agents, to the admixture of biochemical vagaries and so on. Much more study must be undertaken before our understanding is advanced in the area of Reye's syndrome and Reye-like conditions.

The role of aspirin in chronic pain therapy

Peter Evans

Pain Relief Clinic, Charing Cross Hospital, London, UK

INTRODUCTION

One of the problems with chronic pain is that one is looking to some extent at learned behaviour and moving away from a pathogenic process. Thus most therapy is concerned with symptom control (algology). In the pain clinic we see a mixed group of problems (Table 1). The spectrum of conditions includes chronic back pain, those affecting the autonomic pathway, such as sympathetically maintained pain and causalgia, and a variety of less-common problems, such as myofascial pain, and pain associated with degenerative joint disease.

Many patients have suffered pain for prolonged periods and the peak age for presentation is between 50 and 60 years. The primary reason for a referral to a Pain Relief Clinic is because conventional therapy has persistently failed to help relieve symptoms. Almost half the patients will have attended other specialist departments within the hospital and it is hardly surprising that the results of further intervention are poor. In reality, we probably cure <10% of our patients and provide some moderate or long term assistance for a further 35–40%. Most attention is directed to helping patients cope with their pain rather than necessarily relieving all the symptoms. A wide range of therapeutic modalities are employed (Table 2).

Table 1 *Spectrum of conditions—chronic pain patients*

Range of conditions	%	Symptom mean dur	Age years
Chronic back pain	22	9.5	68
Malignancy	11	0.8	62
Autonomic (SMP)	14	5.6	61
Post herpetic	10	4.8	79
Degenerative	9	6.2	68
Post traumatic	9	4.6	46
Peripheral nerve	6	2.9	63
Peripheral vascular	5	4.8	71
Myofascial	3	1.8	38
Trigeminal	2	3.3	61
Atypical facial	2	3.8	55
Unspecified	7	—	—

Aspirin—towards 2000, edited by G. R. Fryers, 1990; Royal Society of Medicine Services International Congress and Symposium Series No. 168, published by Royal Society of Medicine Services Limited.

Table 2 *Chronic back pain (Role of NSAIDs)*
Study design: open—double-blind crossover

	4 h	48 h	7 day	28 day	6 wk	8 wk
Compliance %	100	100	88	58	46	46
No relief %	42	23	3	3	—	—
Slight %	19	38	28	7	—	—
Good %	7	7	32	23	58	50
Complete %	32	32	29	23	42	50

Open study of the use of drug Zomiperac. Patients were given the drug on a six hourly basis for period of one month. They were however free to stop using the drug if no benefit was obtained. In the second month those remaining on the medication entered a double blind study of the active drug versus a placebo.

Therefore when consideration is given to specific analgesic compounds, such as non-steroidal anti-inflammatory drugs (NSAIDs) or aspirin, their effectiveness must be related to the value of all other types of treatment offered to those in chronic pain.

The role of peripherally acting analgesics in chronic pain patients has not been fully evaluated. Often medication has been given on a 'suck it and see' basis. I do not believe that this is good enough in the 1980s. The primary role for aspirin remains the management of mild pain, intermittent pain, mechanical pain and pain associated with an inflammatory process.

LIMITATIONS OF ANALGESIA

One feature that has been noted in the last few years is that not all pain is analgesic-sensitive or more specifically is not sensitive to the effects of the opiates such as morphine. Typical examples of these include the stabbing or shooting pain of trigeminal neuralgia and the burning hypersensitivity associated with post-herpetic neuralgia. Other insensitive conditions include tenesmus and gastric distention. Furthermore it would appear that most of the pains associated with disturbances of the autonomic system are also unresponsive to opiates. However, it has been suggested that in some of these viscerally mediated pains aspirin and similar compounds may have a role to play. Apart from this rather unusual application Aspirin has three principal areas of use. They are in the treatment of cancer pain, in the relief of chronic back pain and in empirical applications of the drug. Furthermore recently interest has been directed towards parenteral applications of the drug with the use of continuous infusions and spinal injections.

When one considers the use of aspirin and other NSAIDs in the management of chronic pain one has to be aware that patients may be expected to take such compounds for considerable periods of time and acceptability of the drug is an important factor. Obvious side effects such as gastrointestinal disturbance are well appreciated but other features such as compliance, tolerance and abuse are less obvious.

Compliance is a real problem. We found from a two-month study that, even when the patients were under close scrutiny, being followed up first at daily and then weekly intervals less than half the patients took the compounds for more than 4–6 weeks (Table 3). This is a problem with any type of analgesic. There is not a direct relationship between the administration of an analgesic and the

Table 3 *Therapeutic modalities*

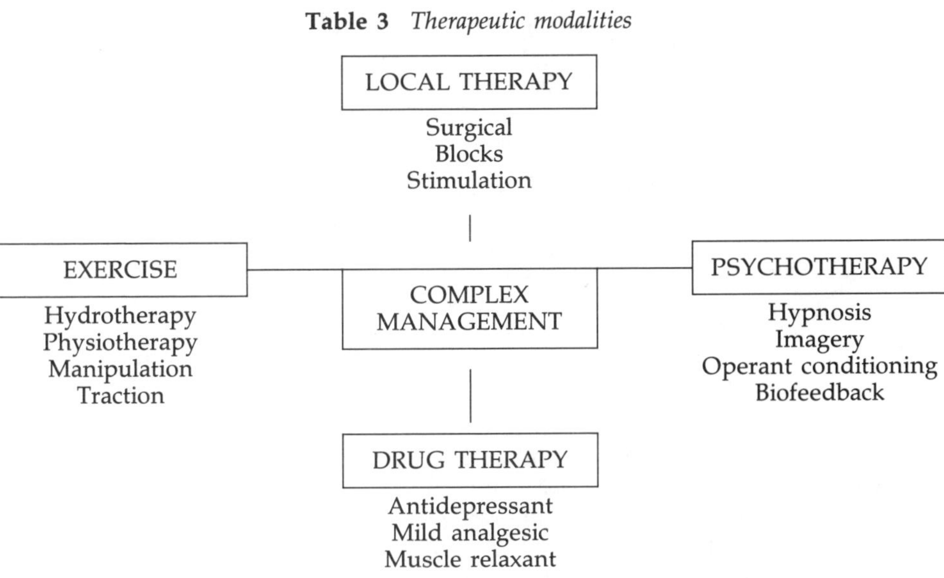

degree, if any, of pain relief that is likely to be achieved. Even if you obtain a therapeutic effect, how do you ensure that your patients will continue to take the medication?

All peripherally acting analgesics exhibit ceiling effects but there is always the potential that patients taking such drugs will try and take more than is necessary to get better effects and so perhaps increase the toxicity and the incidence of side effects. There is a suggestion that perhaps the intrathecal use of peripherally acting compounds may put a different aspect on the situation by producing an additional benefit that could not otherwise be achieved.

A further problem one is likely to observe is that of abuse. By that I do not mean the potential for addiction but certainly many patients with chronic pain use drugs inappropriately. Some will also show abnormal use behaviour with other drugs. These patients often have numerous misconceptions, and part of the psychological management is to re-educate them in the use of medication.

Most believe that more tablets will produce more effect, and many also believe that, if you take them more often, you will again get more effect. One most distressing observation is that some patients will take analgesics because anything is better than nothing, even if little or no analgesia is being obtained. Indeed it is this group who are particularly likely to suffer side-effects from the medication. When we investigated the patients in our clinic, we found that half the patients who were taking non-steroidal and aspirin type medication were not getting any perceived benefit from the drug. Furthermore, a quarter or more of patients were taking more than the recommended upper limit of the medication.

USE IN CHRONIC BACK PAIN

There are many mechanisms said to produce chronic spinal pain (Table 4). Most of them relate to the changes provoked by surgery, such as tissue scarring, the chronic inflammatory state that may occur, and to other problems like arachnoiditis. Even where a plausible process is established the amount of pain that is experienced by the patient may be dependent on many other

Table 4 *Typical causes of chronic back pain*

POST SURGICAL BACK PAIN
Incompletely closed incision
Painful donor site
Fibrosis in muscles
Post surgical instability
Recurrent disc herniation
Continued root pressure from scar tissue
Epidural scarring of multiple nerve roots
Cauda equina syndrome
Facet joint syndrome
Osteoarthritis
Arachnoiditis

unrelated factors. This level of 'current distress' may greatly amplify the pain exhibited by the patient. Ghia and others (1) have suggested that in those patients presenting with chronic low back pain only 15% of the symptoms could be explained by organic disease, and that the rest were due to some other physiological, functional or learned behaviour.

This makes it very difficult to perform useful studies, particularly of analgesics, in this patient group. Whichever analgesic is adopted the outcome is unlikely to be dramatic. One of the major difficulties is trying to assess the severity of pain. Patients use a completely different language in chronic pain as opposed to acute pain; they do not have a stable baseline and the pain is often intermittent in nature. So there are many reasons why, symptomatically, it is very difficult to produce a good study, although that is not a defence for producing no results at all.

When we investigated our back pain patients, we found that 38% of our patients were using aspirin and NSAIDs at the time of presentation. This compared to a 17% prevalence in the total chronic pain population. So clearly there was a patient preference, if nothing else, for these compounds, whether or not there was any significant effect. However, even these results can be misleading. In an open study we conducted of two month's duration, patients received an NSAID (Table 2). In the first few days quite a large number, as expected, failed to derive benefit. As the study continued, a number who obviously did not receive benefit left the study, but we were left with a hard core at the end of the first month of about 25% of our patients who were getting good relief. We then subjected them to a double-blind two-week crossover, and sadly we found at the end of the second month that they really could not tell an active from a placebo agent. So it was likely that the initial benefit was false and it really puts into question the value of short term studies in this patient group.

CANCER PAIN

This is a very emotive area but there are logically very good reasons why one might consider the use of an aspirin-type compound in the management of our patients. Certainly skeletal metastasis would be a primary indication, as would perhaps the use of these drugs in patients with ulceration with or without infection.

Classically, a mechanistic approach is used commencing with the weakest drug and slowly progressing up an analgesic ladder (Table 5) as pain increases

Table 5 *Analgesic ladder*

WEAK non Opiate	Paracetamol—aspirin, nefopam, meptazinol
WEAK OPIATE	Codeine, oxycodone
STRONG OPIATE	Morphine, heroin, methadone, phenazocine, pethidine
STRONG MIXED	Buprenorphine, nalbuphine, pentazocine, butorphanol

in severity. However it should be stressed that even when patients require large doses of opiates it is still rational to continue in tandem the use of aspirin. Both compounds work at different sites and frequently can produce synergistic effects. Even where newer more potent NSAIDs have been produced the benefit is no greater than that achieved from aspirin.

When one investigates the drugs used in the management of patients with malignant disease, one observes that the quality of perceived analgesia is no better with ketoprofen (2) or naproxen (3) than that obtained from aspirin. Unfortunately the use of aspirin alone in the management of cancer pain is rarely adequate and most studies show fall off with time to the extent that after one week less than 30% of patients would be obtaining adequate pain relief. NSAIDs follow a similar pattern. This observation is hardly surprising, the pain of cancer is frequently severe and the limited power of these compounds and their known ceiling effects is bound to limit the scope of their actions.

INTRATHECAL ANALGESIA

Perhaps the most exciting area in pain control that has been developed in the last 10 years is the application of spinally-applied drugs. In 1975 Hughes *et al.* (4) first reported the existence of the endogenous encephalins. From this developed the concept of a variety of specific opiate receptors (5). Further work has suggested that the individual classes of opiate receptor have varied densities in different parts of the central nervous system. For instance the archetypal 'mu' receptor, synonymous with morphine analgesia, has its maximum density in the brain while the 'kappa' receptor appears to have a maximal density in the tissues of the spinal cord. It is therefore conceivable that drugs specific to the spinal cord could produce analgesic effects which were devoid of any of the normal depressant effects of sedation, vomiting and respiratory depression common to all centrally acting analgesics. Furthermore a considerable number of commonly used analgesics have low lipophilicity and in consequence do not easily reach the brain or spinal cord. From the pharmacokinetics it has been estimated that almost 97% of morphine given by the oral or parenteral route does not reach the spinal cord (6) and therefore if it was possible to give the drug peridurally or intrathecally a prolonged and very pronounced effect would be observed. This indeed has been observed (7,8). Since 1980 clinical interest in giving drugs intrathecally has increased and although initial concern was with morphine and other opiate analgesics, Yaksh has indicated that perhaps drugs such as aspirin can have a central effect (9). This is in contrast to previous publications. It has been suggested that NSAIDs may act on receptors for inflammatory mediators, or that they may inhibit multiple functions on membranes and membrane bound enzymes (10). However, Heppelmann *et al.* (11) suggest that aspirin and other NSAIDs have an inhibitory effect on small fibre activity. Using a cat model they studied small group 3 and group 4 unmyelinated afferent nerve fibres coming from an artificially induced arthritic knee joint. They measured both the resting potential in these fibres and also the fibre discharge rate during joint flexion. Then aspirin or indomethacin was administered systemically to the animal and the responses again measured. Ninety minutes after the administration of aspirin, they showed quite clearly that there was a significant reduction, both in the resting and active rates of the firing of these small nerves fibres. This effect was not peculiar to aspirin, a similar response was observed with indomethacin. They further suggested that this inhibition could be reversed by the action of prostaglandin E_2.

This and other work has suggested that aspirin may have a direct neuronal action which could produce a beneficial effect in man if administered intrathecally. It is a relatively benign compound and when injected should not produce any significant side-effects, should not disturb the motor nerves and should not produce respiratory arrest, which is the most serious complication to occur following the administration of intrathecal and peridural opiates.

There are some clinical reports of the use of intrathecal lysine aspirin. However, they are not controlled studies and the results have to be viewed with caution. Pellerin *et al.* (12) demonstrated that in patients with bone pain associated with cancer given doses of between 120 and 720 mg of aspirin, 78% obtained good pain relief. Furthermore the benefit was long lasting. This is an effect that is observed when lipid insoluble opiates are given intrathecally but this can be explained on a reservoir effect. Drugs of low lipid solubility will remain in the CSF and therefore be absorbed into the cord over a long period of time to produce a potentiation effect. However, there is no adequate explanation for the prolonged benefit achieved from aspirin unless some irreversible process was occurring.

A similar study by Devoghel (13) involved a much smaller dose of lysine aspirin (180 mg) mixed with dextrose to produce a 'heavy' spinal solution. Long periods of benefit, as much as 20 days from a single dose were observed, when the results were stratified. Patients with pain associated with cancer had the longest period of relief, those with chronic low back pain had medium periods of relief whilst those with sympathetically maintained pain failed to obtain any benefit.

INTRAVENOUS ANALGESIA

In the United Kingdom it has not been usual to administer aspirin-like compounds intravenously. However a number of reports are suggesting that infusions of lysine aspirin can be effective in relieving postoperative pain. Although ceiling effects may be observed the safety of infusing this drug is clearly advantageous. Jones *et al.* (14) in a double blind study against an infusion of morphine demonstrated that aspirin was equally as effective at controlling the postoperative pain of thoracic surgery. In another study Cashman *et al.* (15) were able to show that as well as equivalent pain relief to morphine being obtained the incidence of sedation, nausea and vomiting was significantly less in the aspirin infusion group. So again, this would appear to be an interesting new application of an old drug.

EMPIRICAL ADMINISTRATION

Over the years a number of empirical applications for aspirin have been found. Recently two reports (16,17) have suggested that topical aspirin may have a role in the management of post-herpetic neuralgia. This condition is typified by the presence of two types of pain. A deep aching sensation associated with cord damage and a more superficial hyperaesthesia and irritation associated with a state of partial denervation. It is for this latter component that aspirin has been applied. A 4% solution of aspirin in chloroform has been used but there are as yet no controlled studies. This is perhaps one of a number of topical preparations that are being considered for this condition, others include capcaicin and vincristin.

REFERENCES

(1) Ghia JN, Duncan G, Toomy TC, Mao W, Greg JM. The pharmacological approach in differential diagnosis of chronic pain. *Spine* 1979; **4**: 4–10.
(2) Turnbull R. Naproxen versus aspirin as analgesics in advanced malignant disease. *J Palliat Care* 1986; **1**: 25–8.
(3) Sacchetti G, Camera P, Rossi AP, Martoni A, Bruni G, Pannuti F. Injectable ketoprofen VS acetylsalicylic acid for the relief of severe cancer pain: double-blind cross-over trial. *Drug Intell Clin Pharm* 1984; **18**: 403–6.
(4) Hughes J, Smith TW, Kosterlitz HW. Isolation of two related pentapeptides from brain with potent opiate activity. *Nature* 1975; **258**: 577–9.
(5) Rance MJ. Multiple opiate receptors—their occurrence and significance. In: Bullingham R, ed. *Opiate analgesia*. Clinics in Anaesthesiology, Vol 1. New York: W B Saunders, 1983: 183–200.
(6) Bullingham RES, McQuay HJ, Moore RA. Extradural and intrathecal narcotics. In: Atkinson RS, Hewer CL, eds. *Recent advances in anaesthesia and analgesia*, 14th Ed. New York: Churchill Livingstone, 1985; **57**: 225–8.
(7) Kotob HI, Hand CW, Moore RA, *et al.*Comparative pharmacokinetics following the intrathecal administration of spinal opiates. *Anaesth Analg* 1986; **65**: 718–22.
(8) Evans PJD, Kotob HIM, Rubin AP. Clinical efficacy of morphine versus diamorphine. *Pain* 1987; **4**(Suppl 70): [Abstract].
(9) Yakash TL. Central and peripheral mechanisms for the antialgesic action of acetylsalicylic acid. In: Barnet HJ, Hirsh M, Mustard JF, eds. *Acetylsalicylic acid: new uses for an old drug*. New York: Raven Press, 1983: 137.
(10) Ferreira SH, Lorenzetti BB, Correa FMA. Central and peripheral action of aspirin like drugs. *Eur J Pharmacol* 1978; **53**: 39–42.
(11) Heppelmann B, Pfeffer HG, Schmidt S, Schmidt RF. Effects of acetylsalicylic acid and indomethacin on single group III and IV sensory units from acutely inflamed joints. *Pain* 1986; **26**: 337–51.
(12) Pellerin M, Hardy F, Abergel A, *et al.* Douleur chronique rebelle des cancereux. *Presse Medicale* 1987; **16**: 1465–8.
(13) Devoghel JC. Small intrathecal doses of lysine acetylsalicylate relieve intractable pain in man. *J Int Med Res* 1983; **11**: 90–1.
(14) Jones RM, Cashman JN, Foster JMG, Wedley JR, Adams AP. Comparison of the infusion of morphine and lysine aspirin for the relief of pain following thoracic surgery. *Br J Anaesthesia* 1988; **57**: 259–63.
(15) Cashman JN, Jones RM, Foster JMG, Adams AP. Comparison of infusions of morphine and lysine aspirin for the relief of pain after surgery. *Br J Anaesthesia* 1985; **57**: 225–8.
(16) King RB. Concerning the management of pain associated with herpes zoster. *Pain* 1988; **33**: 73–8.
(17) Acland RH. A new shingles therapy. *N Z Med J* 1988; **101**: 461.

The role of aspirin in headache

Frederick Frietag

Diamond Headache Clinic, Chicago, USA

INTRODUCTION

In the USA we have undertaken several epidemiological studies on headache, and a number of studies have also taken place in Europe. Up until two weeks ago our best estimates were that there were about 77 million people in the USA who experience tension headache, approximately 35% of the population. Recent studies suggest that these numbers may in fact be far higher, this may be only the tip of the iceberg. Beyond these 77 million people in the USA who experience episodic headache, there are about 45 million people who experience other chronic forms of headache on a more persistent basis and, from an economic viewpoint, this results in a massive amount of lost work days; 156.9 million work days are lost every year in the USA due to chronic headache. The prevalence of migraine runs between 8–20% of the population, so we are looking at a bare minimum of 18 million in the USA alone who experience migraine, and those individuals lose an approximate 64 million work days per year, a large economic toll to be dealt with.

AETIOLOGY

What do we know about headache and its aetiology? First of all there appear to be individuals who never get headache, and others who are more susceptible to it, they carry with them a variety of traits which may make them more prone to the development of headache. They may have alterations in autonomic activity, or of neuroendocrine function, personality characteristics, or even their ability to control pain which may influence the tendency for them to get a headache attack. Outside influences; changes in schedule, weather change, stress, biochemical influences and alterations of biological rhythms may further impact on the likelihood of individuals being susceptible to a headache at a given point in time.

The most prevalent form of headache is the tension headache, or muscle contraction headache, and we know that this is not a homogeneous disorder, it has multiple potential aetiologies. One of the mechanisms felt to be involved in the development of muscle tension headache is an abnormality of stress within the muscles themselves and anxiety may be a factor in creating this. Secondarily there

Aspirin—towards 2000, edited by G. R. Fryers, 1990; Royal Society of Medicine Services International Congress and Symposium Series No. 168, published by Royal Society of Medicine Services Limited.

may also be changes in blood vessel tone, even a vasoconstriction or a vasodilation phenomenon, which is responsible for leading to this sort of headache. Thirdly, in the more chronic, daily constant form of muscle contraction headache, a functional disorder or a biochemical process imbalance, similar to depression, may be responsible.

We see a lot of patients who present with what appear to be muscle contraction type headaches. In examining these individuals it is important to take a careful history and perform a careful examination, since there may be a variety of underlying disorders which may have influencing effects to create headache which would appear to be of the muscle contraction type. Among the disorders that we can see leading to a muscle contraction type headache are disorders of the eye, muscle imbalance, inflammation around the eye itself, sinus infections or other inflammatory conditions of the nose and sinus passages. Viral infections can create a headache which appears to be of a muscle contraction type. In the USA it has become very popular to focus on the role of the temporal mandibular joint as a causative focus of headache; this is overplayed in great part. Disorders of the cervical spine, such as arthritis can create a muscle contraction type headache, and this is well influenced by aspirin. Direct trauma to the scalp or neck muscles with subsequent nerve entrapment in the scar or nerve pinching can create a similar headache. We see patients who experience tumours in the upper neck or the posterior fossa who have a headache which is of a more generalized type, and has all the characteristics of being of muscular origin.

In vascular headaches such as migraine, we see a muscle contraction component at times and this may be an influencing effect on the development of the chronic muscle contraction headache. Life stresses, anxiety, depression, even fibromyalgia may be additional causes of muscle contraction type headaches that have other bases.

Muscle contraction headache takes on a wide variability in its frequency, duration, location and severity. It is an elusive entity. Typically, the headache may have an aching or pressure type of sensation, others will describe it as a squeezing sensation or a heaviness of the head, a tightness or even a weight upon the head. If we look at the range of people who suffer it, we see that approximately 35% of the population from childhood through old age experience it, so it is a disorder throughout all age groups. A study in Denmark (1) investigated some characteristics of the chronic muscle contraction type headache patient. First, there is a great deal of variability in the frequency of occurrence; about half the patients only experience attacks once a month or less. Others may experience it a little more frequently, several times per month, and a much smaller percentage have it on a daily basis. The location of the pain can be the whole head, as it was in about one-third of patients, or it can also be unilateral, as we see occurring in migraine headache more typically. And then a large percentage of patients experience the headache in the forehead, the temple, the occipital region or in variable locations. The pain severity can also be extreme: while many patients' muscle contraction headaches are in the mild range with no incapacitation, a good share of patients in this study had significant headaches that did interfere to some extent with their activities and a small percentage, about 5% of patients, had headaches that were enough to interfere with their regular daily activities. In comparison, a survey by Waters and O'Connor (2) found that a fairly large percentage, 35%, had muscle contraction type headaches which were significant enough to impair their ability to function normally, with a small percentage having relatively insignificant headaches.

One thing we see in a patient who experiences the more chronic daily muscle contraction headache is that there is a higher prevalence of the headache being present in the early morning hours around the time of awakening. Approximately 50% of patients who had muscle contraction headache find the headache present when they wake in the morning, so it is not just a pure tension situation, since they have nothing to be tense about on awakening.

Time of day, or day of onset, of headache has little bearing: it is common throughout the week. For the majority of patients who have muscle contraction headache, the headaches are of brief duration, lasting from less than a few hours to no more than 4 h. Only a small percentage of patients in this study had headaches lasting the majority of the day.

MIXED HEADACHE SYNDROME

In our clinic in Chicago, as in most headache centres, we see the patient who has been unresponsive to a variety of therapies by local physicians or self-help. The most common patient we see is the one who presents with the so-called mixed headache syndrome. It is literally a combination of migraine and a chronic muscle contraction headache occurring together. Mixed headache syndrome goes by a variety of names in the literature; migraine and muscle contraction headache, chronic daily headache, migraine headache with interval headache, the mixed headache syndrome or combined headache. It can take on one of several different presentations. It can occur as a pattern of periodic episodic migraine attacks, very typical in their symptomatology, superimposed on a lower grade but chronic muscle contraction type headache. Other patients will present with a history of increasing frequency of their migraine attacks to the point where they are headachy all the time. Along with this increasing frequency of headache, these patients typically tend to lose the gastrointestinal and neurological symptoms that are the hallmarks of migraine. Thirdly, we see a group of patients whose headaches truly appear to be a blend. They have migraine-type symptomatology, superimposed headaches that are of relatively low intensity but chronic in nature and these are either throbbing or aching and can combine and shift during the course of the day, so they are truly a mixed blend of two distinct pain problems.

Since we may be dealing with two different problems, or problems which interlock with one another, we need to look at some of the factors which predispose the patient to this from a physiological viewpoint. There is a great deal of controversy concerning the pathogenesis of both the muscle contraction headache and migraine; although we have made great strides forward we do not yet have all the answers. Nevertheless, we do have some physiological insights which may help to account for the two disorders.

First of all in migraine, there is often a secondary muscle contraction component that develops as part of the headache process itself. A more generalized headache, more of an aching sensation that often goes into the neck. It is very typical of a muscle contraction type headache as well. There has been a study done by Takashima at Tottori University, Japan (3), who showed that both migraine sufferers and patients with muscle contraction headache, had an abnormality of platelet function: the hypercoagulability that has been suggested as one of the possible mechanisms involved in the genesis of migraine in the past. There may also be a dysregulation of autonomic tone associated with both disorders. Lastly, my partner and trainer in the field of headache, Dr Seymour Diamond in the early 1960s (4) proposed that depression manifests itself as a primary headache

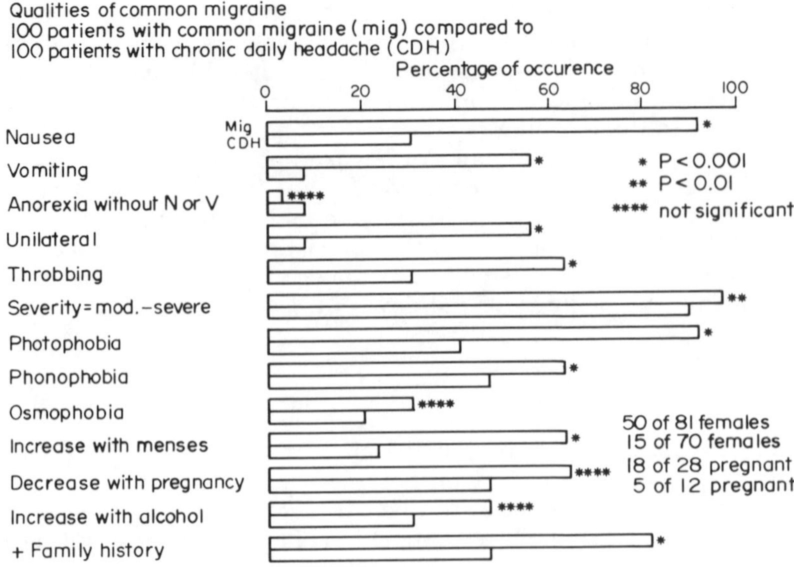

Figure 1 *A comparison between various clinical characteristics in patients with common migraine and patients with tension headache of the chronic daily type. All patients were consecutively seen in a headache clinic. Note that some characteristics have a high, others a low discriminative power. N=nausea, V=vomiting, mod=moderate (Reproduced from* Headache *1988;* ***28****: 124–9, with kind permission).*

disorder that can take on the pattern of both migraine or the chronic muscle contraction headache or both. So we have several possible interlinking mechanisms.

In patients who have mixed headache, we see from a study by Solomon and Kaplan in New York (5) (Fig. 1), that a good share of patients who had chronic daily headache had migrainous symptoms such as nausea or vomiting; it was not as common as is seen in those patients with pure common migraine, but still a large percentage did experience typical gastrointestinal symptoms related to migraine. The pain severity did not differ substantially between the two disorders and many of the patients had either unilateral headache or a throbbing headache which is now used as part of the diagnostic requirements for the current diagnosis of migraine using the classification from the International Headache Society.

Pregnancy typically ameliorates migraine as it did chronic daily headache in many patients, not just the migrainous component but even the daily muscle contraction component. So these two disorders may have some common links.

THERAPY AND THE ROLE OF ASPIRIN

Turning to therapy and the role of aspirin in the treatment of headache, Seymour Diamond did a study several years ago (6) (Table 1), looking at the beneficial effects of aspirin vs ibuprofen vs placebo in a parallel study where the patients were being treated for tension headaches. From the data one sees that the patients all experienced relatively moderate levels of pain and that 3 h after taking the medication the three active treatment groups did receive a substantial reduction in their pain as compared to the placebo-treated group. We see from these values

Table 1 *Ibuprofen versus aspirin and placebo in the treatment of muscle contraction headache*

Treatment Group	Mean PID Score	Mean SPID Score	Mean Maximum PID Score	Mean Minimum PID Score
Ibuprofen 400 mg	0.81 (p=0.018)	3.24	1.24	0.38
Ibuprofen 800 mg	0.91 (p=0.002)	3.63	1.50 (p=0.019)	0.33
Aspirin 650 mg	0.90 (p=0.002)	3.50	1.50 (p=0.013)	0.33
Placebo	0.55	2.05	0.91	0.09

that the results for aspirin 650 mg, dropping from 2.96 to 2.13, are not substantially different from those achieved with ibuprofen 800 mg—2.86 to 1.99. They actually appeared to be somewhat better than using ibuprofen 400 mg. Examining the pain intensity difference scores, and their changes, three active treatment groups showed a significant improvement compared to placebo in a mean pain intensity difference score. And when we look again we see that for ibuprofen 400 mg vs aspirin, while both were significant, there was more substantive reduction than for ibuprofen. When aspirin is compared with the 800 mg dose of ibuprofen nearly identical results are seen.

A group from the University of Texas, led by Peters (7) (Fig. 2), examined the use of aspirin 650 mg vs paracetamol 1000 mg vs placebo in both tension and tension-vascular headache, and up to the 5–6 h point aspirin and paracetamol at those dosages did provide significant reductions in the pain testing scores.

Pain control was one of the factors that influenced headache outcome. In the first 3 h, aspirin produced better results than paracetamol, and this is important because, if we can stop the pain more quickly, we are more likely to get a more favourable outcome with complete amelioration of the headache than if

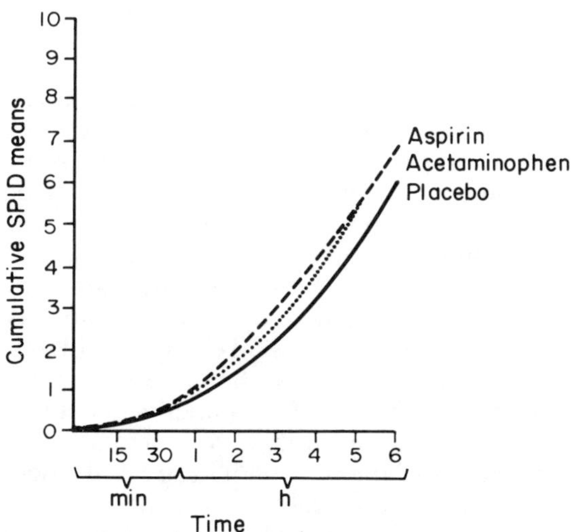

Figure 2 *Cumulative sums of pain intensity difference (SPID) means in 162 subjects with tension-vascular type headaches. (Reproduced from* American Journal of Medicine *1983; 285: 36–42, with kind permission).*

we allow the headache to drag on, requiring progressively increasing doses of analgesic agents.

In summary, aspirin is certainly superior to placebo in straight tension headache, it is comparable and possibly superior to paracetamol 1000 mg, it appears to be superior to ibuprofen 400 mg and at least comparable to ibuprofen 800 mg. So a relatively small dose can provide significant results in tension headache, compared with other agents.

TREATMENT AT THE DIAMOND HEADACHE CLINIC

In our clinic our intractable patients have been everywhere and seen everyone. The average patient has had headaches on a daily basis for 20 years, has sought advice from six physicians and taken an average of 12 prescription medications, plus a host of over-the-counter preparations in attempts to relieve their pain, but still they end up on our doorstep and we are asked to help solve their problem. These patients are not easy to control, requiring a balanced regimen of medications and other non-drug therapies in order to help provide them with substantial relief of their headaches. Most of these patients, when they come to us, have become habituated to either narcotics, barbiturates or to caffeine-containing analgesics or coffee, tea or soft drinks. These have a detrimental effect on their headaches.

We treat these patients aggressively, we detoxify them in our inpatient unit and when we send them home, approximately 90% of them leave our unit utilizing a salicylate aspirin derivative, choline salicylate, as their sole analgesic for the majority of their subsequent headaches that they may continue to experience in the early stages of treatment. We have approximately 90% success rate from our inpatient unit, so a large percentage of patients can utilize a very simple preparation of an aspirin derivative for their treatment. One of the reasons we make use of this aspirin derivative is that we are dealing with a jaded patient as well. They have had their headaches for a long time, they have taken everything and, even though we may be their last hope, we still have to deal with their psyche, which tells them that they have these terrible headaches which require these strong narcotic analgesics to control their pain, and now they are told to control the headache with aspirin. That is a public relations problem that we have to confront, and we use the aspirin derivative. Many of our patients make the switch from this liquid preparation to straight aspirin-containing tablets because they are more convenient and they find them to be of equal efficacy as their headaches continue to remit and they gain confidence in their ability to control their headaches with simple analgesic preparations.

Some interesting research has been done with the aspirin derivative lysine aspirin by Fukuda and Izumikawa (8) from Japan, using an intravenous preparation. They treated patients who had combined migraine/muscle contraction headaches and six of their patients had favourable outcomes. Within 20 min of administration of lysine aspirin two of the patients had an almost entire remission of their acute headache and an additional four had at least a partial response to this preparation. In many of these patients the headaches had been prolonged over a course of days and so to get relief within 20 min was rather dramatic. This group from Japan suggest that in trigeminal neuralgia lysine aspirin may provide significant relief of the acute episode, so we may need to look at this in more detail as we get better understanding of a presumed central action of what were previously believed to be peripherally-acting analgesics.

CONCLUSIONS

In summary, the patient who has a difficult headache problem requires first of all a safe and effective analgesic for the relief of their headache. If they have headaches on a daily or nearly daily basis the use of narcotics or barbiturates are certainly contraindicated, as they are habituating and, from our work and from the work of others, we see that aspirin or an aspirin derivative can provide substantial relief of the acute headache for the vast majority of individuals. This is especially so when it is combined with appropriate other medical therapies for reduction of the frequency and severity of the attacks, utilizing medications such as antidepressants and β-blockers for the migraine and the muscle contraction type headaches, physical modalities, muscle relaxants as adjuvants, biofeedback and counselling. We do not utilize tranquillizers in most patients unless they have a chronic anxiety disorder which is unresponsive in the early stages to counselling.

So aspirin is a good analgesic, it works well in headache, and there is much room to conduct further research and to develop new products such as lysine aspirin as effective therapies for headache.

REFERENCES

(1) Hollnagel H, Nrrelund N. Headache in 40 year old persons in Glostrup, Denmark. *Ugeskr, haeg* 1980; **142**: 3071–7.
(2) Waters WE, O'Connor PJ. Epidemiology of headache and migraine in women. *J Neurol Neurosurg Psychiatry* 1971; **34**: 148–53.
(3) Takeshima T, Takao Y, Urakami K, Nishikawa S, Takahashi K. Muscle contraction headache and migraine. Platelet activation and plasma norepinephrine during the cold pressor test. *Cephalalgia* 1989; **9**: 7–13.
(4) Diamond S. Depressive headaches. *Headache* 1964; **4**: 255–9.
(5) Solomon S, Kappa KG, Smith CR. Common migrain: criteria for diagnosis. *Headache* 1988; **28**: 124–9.
(6) Diamond S. Ibuprofen versus aspirin and placebo in the treatment of muscle contraction headache. *Headache* 1983; **23**: 206–10.
(7) Peters BH, Fraim CJ, Masel BE. Comparison of 650 mg aspirin and 1,000 mg acetaminophen with each other and with placebo in moderately severe headache. *Am J Med* 1983; **285**: 36–42.
(8) Fukuda Y, Izumikawa K. Intravenous aspirin for intractable headache and facial pain. *Headache* 1988; **28**: 47–50.

Aspirin and migraine

Paul Davies

Department of Neurology, Charing Cross Hospital, London, UK

An acute migraine attack is recognized by its characteristic pattern of symptoms. There may be vague non-focal neurological symptoms such as elation, depression or hunger during the 24 h before the onset proper, then the focal neurological symptoms of the aura which are usually visual but may include disturbance of speech, hemianaesthesia or rarely hemiparesis. The headache, often the most severe symptom of the attack, is usually unilateral, severe and throbbing and may be associated with nausea and vomiting, photophobia, phonophobia and osmophobia. The symptomatology of migraine is both complex and varied but the assessment of drug efficacy in acute treatment has usually only considered effects on headache, nausea and vomiting or effects on overall function of daily activities.

Aspirin has been shown to be useful in the acute and prophylactic treatment of migraine. The main pharmacological action of aspirin is cyclo-oxygenase inhibition, thereby inhibiting prostaglandin production throughout the body. It is not clear how prostaglandins are involved in the production of migraine symptoms. A trigger factor or factors may often be identified but little is known how or indeed where a migraine attack is initiated. Attention has focused on the brain, the cranial vasculature as well as the circulating blood platelets in an attempt to generate hypotheses of migraine pathogenesis. Aspirin, and other non-steroidal anti-inflammatory drugs (NSAIDs), are well known for their inhibitory action on platelet aggregation but the role of the platelet in migraine symptom production is uncertain. Platelets of migraine sufferers are hyperaggreggable and there is a platelet release reaction during a migraine attack but the severity of the attack bears no relation to the concentration of platelet release products which can be measured in the circulation during the attack. At present, most migraine specialists consider that migraine is primarily a neuronal disturbance but that the cranial vasculature is involved in at least the headache phase of the attack. The occurrence of a sterile inflammatory process surrounding extracranial blood vessels during the headache phase of the attack is generally accepted. Algetic substances (e.g. serotonin and prostaglandins) in the sterile inflammation sensitize the pain fibres which carry pain information to the central nervous system. Pain control is complex and it is known that in the spinal cord there are descending as well as ascending pain modulating pathways and that serotonin, encephalins and prostaglandins may act at various levels to control pain transmission. Aspirin may well have a central action in pain modulation.

Aspirin—towards 2000, edited by G. R. Fryers, 1990; Royal Society of Medicine Services International Congress and Symposium Series No. 168, published by Royal Society of Medicine Services Limited.

Several substances have been infused into volunteers to see whether migraine attacks could be initiated. Carlsson (1) injected prostaglandin E1 (PGE_1), a hyperalgetic agent, into normal volunteers and found that he could produce bilateral headache in seven out of eight subjects. Peatfield at the Princess Margaret Migraine Clinic, infused prostacyclin into migraine patients and into controls and was unable to induce migraine in migraine sufferers, although some experienced headache this was no greater in migraine subjects than in controls (2).

Clinical trials to evaluate aspirin and other non-steroidal anti-inflammatory drugs effective in the acute treatment of migraine are beset by methodological problems. Firstly the question of case definition may not be exactly stated, symptoms are subjective and difficult if not impossible to quantify. Migraine sufferers experience other types of headache and they often cannot distinguish the start of a migraine attack from the start of another type of headache e.g. tension headache. Those with frequent headaches commonly abuse analgesics and over frequent use can lead to analgesic headaches. During a migraine attack there is impaired drug absorption by the oral route so that other routes of administration or a combination with an anti-emetic must be considered. We also know that there is a large placebo effect with maybe 30–40% of patients responding favourably to placebo.

ASPIRIN AND ACUTE MIGRAINE TREATMENT

Aspirin can be considered within the family of non-steroidal anti-inflammatory drugs in acute migraine treatment. From clinical experience sodium diclophenac (75 mg) intramuscularly is one of the most effective acute migraine treatments. It is the only NSAID that can be administered by that route. Naproxen, ibuprofen, ketoprofen, mefenamic acid and tolfenamic acid have all been found effective in acute migraine treatment. Interestingly, indomethacin has not been found to be effective—headache is a common side effect with this drug.

The first study of aspirin in acute migraine treatment carried out in a scientific manner was by Ross-Lee (3). In a retrospective study of 61 patients he found that soluble aspirin usually, or always, relieved migraine attacks in 44% of patients and sometimes relieved the disorder in another 25%. Adverse effects were reported in 16%, mainly nausea and vomiting, which was probably due to the attack itself. The response to aspirin was unrelated to the patient's age, or duration of migraine history. Surprisingly, he found that the response was not related to the severity of the migraine attack or the occurrence of nausea and vomiting. The presence of an aura appeared to improve the chance of a response to aspirin; presumably patients were able to treat their attacks at an earlier stage.

Volans, when he was a Migraine Trust research registrar, studied the absorption of 900 mg of effervescent aspirin during an acute migraine attack in 42 patients and 20 controls (4). Nineteen of the patients showed significant impairment of aspirin absorption which correlates with the severity of the headache and with the gastrointestinal symptoms at the time of treatment but not with the duration of the attack or migraine type. Nausea and/or vomiting are almost universal in migraine attacks and we know from barium meal studies that gastric dilatation occurs at this time. Volans proceeded to look at the effect of metoclopramide on the absorption of effervescent aspirin in acute and asymptomatic migraine sufferers and in normal controls (5). One group of migraineurs was given effervescent aspirin only, 900 mg, and a second group then received intramuscular metoclopramide, 10 mg, 10 min before the same dose of aspirin. During a migraine attack, and after aspirin alone, there was a significant impairment in the rate of aspirin absorption compared to headache free migraineurs or normal volunteers. With intramuscular metoclopramide treatment, absorption became similar to normal volunteers.

Ross-Lee, several years later, compared the absorption, in acute migraine attacks, of soluble aspirin alone and in combination with oral or intramuscular metoclopramide (6). Higher peak aspirin levels occurred with the addition of oral or intramuscular metclopramide. Aspirin appeared earlier in the plasma with oral metoclopramide and there was better early pain relief. By 1 h from dosing intramuscular metoclopramide was also associated with better pain relief than aspirin alone. Tfelt-Hansen and Olesen compared metoclopramide (10 mg) and aspirin (650 mg) in effervescent formulation (Migravess®) with effervescent aspirin (650 mg, Alka Seltzer®) or placebo in a double-blind study of 118 migraine sufferers (7). Eighty-five patients completed all three forms of treatment. Aspirin was significantly better than placebo for pain relief, but not quite significant for nausea relief whereas Migravess was significantly better than placebo for pain and nausea relief but there was no significant difference between aspirin and the combination with regard to analgesic or antiemetic effects. They considered that the dose of metoclopramide was probably too low in this preparation.

Brandon *et al.* looked at a new, pleasant-tasting formulation of aspirin, glycinated aspirin, in normal healthy volunteers and assessed the bioavailability of this aspirin preparation when given in a variety of ways; swallowed with 200 ml of water, dissolved sublingually and retained in the mouth, or dispersed on the tongue and swallowed without water (8). There was no detectable absorption of aspirin when retained in the mouth but equal absorption when swallowed with or without water. They found no difference in efficacy when the glycinated aspirin was swallowed with or without water during an acute migraine attack.

Intravenous aspirin has been used for pain relief in a variety of conditions. Noda *et al.* (9) reported on its beneficial effects in three patients with severe acute migraine attacks. Intravenous aspirin (DL-lysine-acetyl-salicylate, Venoprin®) has been available in Japan since 1983. One vial contains 497 mg of aspirin. They report that about 15 min after the injection in three patients 'the headache disappeared completely without any side-effect'. Aspirin treatment of acute migraine attacks has been compared with several other acute treatments. In 1980 Tfelt-Hansen and Olesen compared aspirin with paracetamol in a double blind trial (10). At that time their standard treatment for acute migraine attacks at their clinic was metoclopramide 10 mg im, diazepam 5 mg orally and then aspirin 1 g orally or paracetamol 1 g orally. From their study of 600 patients they concluded that aspirin and paracetamol were of equal efficacy.

ASPIRIN AND MIGRAINE PROPHYLAXIS

O'Neill and Mann carried out a double-blind crossover study of aspirin 650 mg twice a day against placebo in 12 patients (11). The criteria for the diagnosis of migraine were not exactly stated. Treatment was for three months with each agent and in seven patients platelet aggregation to epinephrine and adenosine diphosphate was studied during the trial. In nine patients with aspirin treatment a highly significant reduction in headache frequency was seen, all the responders were those with classical migraine, all the females in the study responded and those with hyperaggreggable platelets seemed to respond best of all. Following the idea that platelet aggregation inhibition was an important mechanism in migraine prophylaxis, Masel *et al.* (12), in a double-blind crossover study, compared aspirin 325 mg twice a day combined with dipyridamole 25 mg three times a day against placebo in 25 patients. The active treatment was significantly better than placebo with 68% of patients reporting subjective improvement while on active treatment.

In 1981, Ryan and Ryan considered they had a new approach to migraine prophylaxis and carried out a double-blind parallel group study (13). There were 40 patients in each of four groups, one group received dipyridamole 75 mg four times a day; another group aspirin 325 mg four times a day; and another group dipyridamole 75 mg plus aspirin 325 mg four times a day while the fourth group received placebo. They concluded that the best reduction in attack frequency and severity was with aspirin and dipyridamole combined but that both aspirin alone and dipyridamole alone were better than placebo.

The optimum dose of aspirin for migraine prophylaxis is uncertain. Wind and Punt advocate low-dose aspirin (60–80 mg/day) and have provided some evidence in support of this claim (14,15). Peto *et al.* in a randomized trial of prophylactic daily aspirin among British male doctors, allocated two thirds of the subjects effervescent or soluble aspirin 500 mg each day (or 300 mg enteric coated aspirin if subsequently requested) while one third were asked to avoid aspirin, there was no placebo group (16). There was a highly significant decrease in the reporting of migraine attacks in the aspirin-treated group. They suggested that more work was needed to assess the efficacy of aspirin in migraine prophylaxis.

Baldrati *et al.* in a small study compared aspirin with the 'gold standard' in migraine prophylaxis, propranolol (17). They cautiously suggested that aspirin was equally as effective as propranolol.

ASPIRIN, PLATELETS AND MIGRAINE PROPHYLAXIS

In recent years the platelet theory of migraine pathogenesis has come into disrepute. In testing this theory one approach has been to give daily aspirin, assess platelet aggregation in time and try to correlate change in aggregation with clinical outcome. Smith *et al.* studied 46 patients, each taking aspirin 250 mg each day for two months and 10 controls (18). Platelet aggregation was measured during the study. They concluded that the results confirmed platelet hyperaggregability in migraine patients, a reduction of aggregation was seen with aspirin treatment but there was no evidence of any significant clinical improvement, thus falsifying the hypothesis of migraine as a platelet aggregation disorder.

Along similar lines, Hosman-Benjaminse and Bolhuis studied aspirin 160 mg each day in 27 migraine patients in a double-blind, placebo-controlled crossover study in which patients had three months of each treatment (19). There was no correlation between migraine attacks and aspirin effects on ADP-induced platelet aggregation and no difference in efficacy between aspirin and placebo.

Further evidence that platelet aggregation inhibition is unimportant for migraine prophylaxis comes from studies with dipyridamole. It may be useful in low dosage (100 mg/day) but higher doses may actually provoke migraine (20).

CONCLUSIONS

There is good evidence that aspirin is effective acute treatment for migraine but its precise mode of action is unclear. As with all acute migraine treatment, unless there is adequate drug absorption there will be little or no clinical benefit.

Combined with metoclopramide, higher levels of aspirin are achieved and there is subsequently greater clinical response. Other routes of aspirin administration have been studied, intravenous aspirin appears to be an area in which further research may prove useful.

For migraine prophylaxis, aspirin at high dose (650 mg/day) appears to be effective. Benefit does not necessarily follow from an inhibition of platelet aggregation.

Although the pharmaceutical industry appears to have new and exciting treatments for migraine on the horizon we would do well to remember the words of Professor Matthews in his book on *Practical Neurology* (21).

'It is a frequent and rather humiliating experience to be told that after all the most recently introduced ergotamine preparations have failed, that a couple of aspirins seem to do the trick'.

REFERENCES

(1) Carlsson LA, Eklund LG, Oro L. Clinical and metabolic effects of different doses of PGE_1 in man. *Acta Med Scand* 1968; **183**: 423–30.

(2) Peatfield RC, Gavel MJ, Clifford F. The effect of infused prostacyclin in migraine and cluster headache. *Headache* 1981; **21**: 190–5.

(3) Ross-Lee L, Eadie MJ, Tyrer JH. Aspirin treatment of migraine attacks: clinical observations. *Cephalalgia* 1982; **2**: 71–6.

(4) Volans GN. Absorption of effervescent aspirin during migraine. *BMJ* 1974; **4**: 265–9.

(5) Volans GN. The effect of metoclopramide on the absorption of effervescent aspirin in migraine. *Br J Clin Pharmacol* 1975; **2**: 57–63.

(6) Ross-Lee LM, Heazlewood V, Tyrer JH, Eadie MJ. Aspirin treatment of migraine attacks: plasma drug level data. *Cephalalgia* 1982; **2**: 9–14.

(7) Tfelt-Hansen P, Olesen J. Effervescent metoclopramide and aspirin (Migravess®) versus effervescent aspirin or placebo for migraine attacks: a double-blind study. *Cephalalgia* 1984; **4**: 107–11.

(8) Brandon RA, Eadie MJ, Curran ACW, Nolan PC, Presneill JJ, Patterson MC. A new formulation of aspirin: bioavailability and analgesic efficacy in migraine attacks. *Cephalalgia* 1986; **6**(1): 19–27.

(9) Noda S, Itoh H, Umezaki H. Successful treatment of migraine attacks with intravenous injection of aspirin. *J Neurol Neurosurg Psychiatry* 1985; **48**(11): 1187.

(10) Tfelt-Hansen P, Olesen J. Paracetamol (acetaminophen) versus acetylsalicylic acid in migraine. *Eur Neurol* 1980; **19**: 163–5.

(11) O'Neil BP, Mann JD. Aspirin prophylaxis in migraine. *Lancet* 1978; **ii**: 1179–81.

(12) Masel BE, Chesson Al, Peters BH, Levin HS, Alperin JB. Platelet antagonists in migraine prophylaxis. A clinical trial using aspirin and dipyridamole. *Headache* 1980; **20**: 13–18.

(13) Ryan RE, Ryan RE. Migraine prophylaxis: a new approach. *Laryngoscope* 1981; **91**: 1501–6.

(14) Wind J, Punt J. Low dose aspirin and migraine prophylaxis. *Laryngoscope* 1982; **92**: 1198–9.

(15) Wind J, Punt J. Migraine prophylaxis with low-dose aspirin: a promising new approach. In: Rose FC, ed. *New advances in headache research*. London: Smith Gordon 1989.

(16) Peto R, Gray R, Collins R, *et al.* Randomised trial of prophylactic daily aspirin in British male doctors. *BMJ* 1988; **296**: 313–16.

(17) Baldrati A, Cortelli P, Procaccianti G, *et al.* Propranolol and acetylsalicyclic acid in migraine prophylaxis. Double-blind cross over study. *Acta Neurol Scand* 1983; **67**(3): 181–6.

(18) Smith M, Jerusalem F, Rhyner K, Isler H. Salicylate prophylaxis in migrane. *Schweiz Arch Neurol Neurochir Psychiatry* 1984; **135**(2): 273–5.
(19) Hosman-Benjaminse SL, Bolhuis PA. Migraine and platelet aggregation in patients treated with low dose ASA. *Headache* 1986; **26**: 282–4.
(20) Hawkes CH. Dipyridamole in migraine. *Lancet* 1978; **ii**: 153.
(21) Matthews WB. *Practical neurology*. Oxford: Blackwell, 1963.

The aetiology of analgesic nephropathy

D. N. S. Kerr

Royal Postgraduate Medical School, The Hammersmith Hospital, London, UK

EFFECTS OF ASPIRIN ON THE KIDNEY

Tubular cell excretion and enzymuria

A number of effects of aspirin on the kidney have been described; the acute effects were reviewed in detail in a previous Aspirin Symposium (1). The phenomenon of acute shedding of renal tubular cells was described in the early part of the present century (reviewed by Prescott (2)). A more recent study by Burry and Colleagues (3) showed that renal tubular cell excretion rises rapidly over the first few days and then falls back over about 10 days to the baseline level of excretion suggesting that the acute proximal tubular insult is short-lived. Enzyme excretion continues for at least two weeks and is present in some patients for as long as they take aspirin (3). However, it seems an entirely reversible change in renal function.

Change in glomerular filtration rate (GFR) and renal plasma flow (RPF)

In normal subjects aspirin infusion causes a fall in GFR and RPF (4,5). However, when aspirin is given orally in normal therapeutic doses the only changes usually found are a rise in serum creatinine and a fall in creatinine clearance (6). These are probably due to the effect of aspirin on the transport of substances like creatinine in the renal tubule; the lack of any effect on true GFR is indicated by stable plasma urea and slight, usually insignificant, changes in more reliable measures of GFR such as ethylenediaminetetra-acetic acid (EDTA) clearance. Other human studies were reviewed by Kerr (1); in summary they indicate that aspirin depresses GFR and renal plasma flow by a modest amount in normal subjects exposed to intravenous infusion, very high oral doses and simultaneous sodium depletion but has little or no effect on GFR in normal therapeutic doses.

A much more pronounced effect on GFR is observed in patients with systemic lupus erythematosus (SLE) and other diseases causing glomerulonephritis. It has been particularly well studied and described by Kimberley and Plotz from the National Institutes of health in the USA (7–10). They found that as serum salicylate levels rose to the therapeutic range, during treatment of the arthralgia of SLE, there was a simultaneous rise in serum creatinine, a fall in creatinine clearance and a rise in blood urea, confirming that this was a true change in GFR. These changes

Aspirin—towards 2000, edited by G. R. Fryers, 1990; Royal Society of Medicine Services International Congress and Symposium Series No. 168, published by Royal Society of Medicine Services Limited.

were accompanied by a reduced excretion of prostaglandin metabolites; the suggestion of Kimberley and Plotz that aspirin caused these changes in renal function by inhibition of prostaglandin synthetase has not been challenged. The same mechanism has been invoked to explain the reduction in proteinuria in nephrotic syndrome (11) and the antagonism of diuretic action (12) by aspirin and other cyclo-oxygenase inhibitors.

Acute renal failure

The depression of GFR caused by aspirin in glomerulonephritis is usually modest but occasionally amounts to mild acute renal failure (13); it is rapidly reversible on withdrawal of the drug. More severe accute renal failure has been recorded very rarely in two circumstances. Acute interstitial nephritis has been described in a handful of cases as part of a general hypersensitivity reaction, such as occurs much more frequently with other non-steroidal anti-inflammatory agents, notably fenoprofen (14). Acute renal failure after self-poisoning must be very rare—I encountered only one patient in 25 years on the renal unit in Newcastle-upon-Tyne during a period when aspirin was one of the commonest agents used in self-poisoning; he had ingested over 30 g of aspirin. Campbell and Maclaurin (15) described one patient with acute renal failure following ingestion of 25 g of aspirin and found three previous cases in a search of the literature. However, their conclusion that 'renal damage in salicylate poisoning may be commoner than is generally appreciated' has not been borne out by subsequent experience. There was only one death in acute renal failure among 97 patients with plasma levels over 700 mg/l in the Edinburgh series (16).

THE ROLE OF ASPIRIN IN ANALGESIC NEPHROPATHY

Diagnosing the disease

At a symposium on analgesic nephropathy in London in 1985 Nancy Dreyer, an American epidemiologist from Massachusetts, cast doubt on its existence, ccommenting 'christening a disease by its putative cause may have misled researchers into believing that the evidence for the association has withstood vigorous testing' (17). I beg to differ; I do not think there is a nephrologist in Belgium, where this is a common disease (18), who doubts that he can diagnose analgesic nephropathy at the stage of renal failure. Recognizing it early in its course, and determining the risk associated with different levels of analgesic consumption are different matters that continue to tax the minds of nephrologists and epidemiologists (19). In this presentation I describe the disease as seen in a typical British patient; fuller reviews of the clinical radiological and histological features have been presented elsewhere (20–22).

Patient 1 was a 40 year old woman who presented with acute renal failure (plasma urea 80 mmol/l) after about 15 years consuming mixed analgesics during which time she took about 8 kg phenacetin, 8 kg aspirin and assorted additives including codeine and caffeine. Following haemodialysis and rehydration her GFR rose to about 14 ml/min. She remained in stable chronic renal failure for the next 10 years before suffering a slow decline into terminal renal failure, requiring regular dialysis. Prolonged preservation of renal function after withdrawal of analgesic intake is characteristic of analgesic nephropathy and is the main reason for seeking the diagnosis diligently among patients with 'chronic renal failure, cause unknown' (23–25). However, this patient was unusual in surviving so long at a low GFR; patients with analgesic nephropathy suffer from progressive focal sclerosis if their renal function mass is sufficiently reduced, as do those with any other form of chronic renal disease (26,27), so renal survival is determined by the amount of renal tissue functioning after treatment of aggravating factors such as dehydration and urinary infection (28). However, continuing consumption of analgesics, or relapse to addiction, is the major cause of rapid decline in renal function during follow-up (29); it was detected once in her but stopped in time to prevent serious loss of renal function.

She had a psychiatric history including barbiturate addiction, she had anaemia out of proportion to the severity of her renal failure and she developed a gastric ulcer with melaena, all well-recognized features of analgesic over-consumption. She took her pills for headache which has been the commonest reason for analgesic abuse in almost every published account. She had hypertriglyceridaemia and hypercholesterolaemia; these are features of chronic renal failure of any type but are particularly characteristic of analgesic nephropathy (30) and are a presumed cause of the increased incidence of atheroma which has been reported from Australia (26,31) though not from all countries (32).

Peptic ulcer, from which she suffered, is a common feature of this disease in those countries where aspirin is a major component of analgesic mixtures; it is attributed to the high intake of aspirin, higher than is ever used therapeutically. Hypertension, from which she also suffered, is another common complication affecting about 50% of patients in large published series. Her final decline in renal function was hastened by the use of ergocalciferol to treat her renal bone disease in the years before alfacalcidol and calcitriol became available. Bone disease is common in analgesic nephropathy and is often of the unusual osteomalacic variety which is associated with renal diseases that cause acidosis (33); in one Australian study 14/15 patients developed osteomalacia compared with 2/15 controls with other chronic renal diseases (34). My patient exhibited this tendency to acidosis and required medication with sodium bicarbonate which exacerbated her hypertension. Despite this she passed through two episodes of acute sodium depletion, which is another well-recognized feature of the disease. She suffered from urinary infections and between attacks she had persistent sterile pyuria. Both are common features of analgesic nephropathy which in some published series have affected 100% of patients. In countries like Belgium, analgesic nephropathy is a much commoner cause of sterile pyuria than tuberculosis.

My patient had a symptom complex which, taken together, clinicians recognize as typical of analgesic nephropathy but none of these features is specific to the disease and many are found in chronic renal failure of other causes, so it is seldom possible to make a definite diagnosis on clinical findings alone. The urinary findings are also rather non-specific: slight proteinuria, sterile pyuria, a few granular casts and a pronounced deficit in concentrating and acidifying capacity for the level of GFR.

The feature which is most diagnostic is the occurrence of papillary necrosis which has been the keystone of diagnosis in all autopsy series. Sometimes one can make a histological diagnosis in life because the patient passes a necrotic papilla in the urine. More often, however, one must seek the characteristic radiological findings: the ring sign of contrast surrounding a sloughed papilla; the cavitated papillae from which the sloughs have already passed; the sinus alongside a partially separated papilla; calcified papillae; obstruction of a ureter by a radiolucent sloughed papilla; the presence of renal calculi with radiolucent centres which have formed around sloughed papillae. However, these diagnostic signs are found in only a minority of the patients in whom we diagnose analgesic nephropathy. In the remainder the kidneys appear normal on IVU or show changes which are not distinguishable from those of chronic pyelonephritis.

Reports from Germany have averred that ultrasonic diagnosis of calcified papillae is a more sensitive test for analgesic nephropathy than its radiological equivalents, at least at the stage of renal failure (35,36). So far there is little literature from elsewhere on this test but the illustrations in the original articles are impressive. However, it is unlikely to prove of much value in early diagnosis.

Papillary necrosis has causes other than analgesic nephropathy so its diagnostic significance is not absolute. In a centre like Sydney with a very high incidence of analgesic nephropathy a finding of papillary necrosis papillary necrosis was due to analgesics in 47 of 50 cases (37) whereas in Nottingham, an area of low incidence, analgesic nephropathy was ranked third, after diabetes and urinary obstruction, as a cause of papillary necrosis at autopsy (38). There is, therefore, a need for an alternative diagnostic criterion, preferably one which is present earlier in the disease. The only candidate is capillary sclerosis. This is easily recognized on electron microscopy which shows immense concentric thickening of the capillary wall. When found it is almost pathognomonic of analgesic nephropathy. In the studies of Mihatsch, who first described capillary sclerosis, it was found in 83% of all patients with analgesic nephropathy but in only 3.5% of control autopsies (39). However, it is typically found in the renal pelvis and around the ureters which are not sites readily accessible to biopsy. It affects the bladder in a minority of patients in life and the site which yields the most positive results is the trigone which is an uncomfortable site for biopsy. Analgesic nephropathy is not unique among diseases in lacking a single diagnostic test which is 100% sensitive and specific; in practice the diagnosis can usually be made with considerable confidence by a combination of clinical assessment, imaging and histology. My reply to Nancy Dreyer is 'analgesic nephropathy is alive and well and has been seen in Belgium'.

CAUSES OF ANALGESIC NEPHROPATHY

Phenacetin was once considered the only culprit and the condition was called 'phenacetin nephropathy' but this is clearly a misnomer. Many different non-steroidal analgesics can produce the lesion in animals. At least 18 have been incriminated in man and almost 200 case reports have been collected by Prescott (2) in which patients had taken drugs other than phenacetin. But is phenacetin the major culprit? Many authors, including myself, believe the answer is 'yes', both because it has been the common ingredient in most reports, and because the incidence of analgesic nephropathy has fallen in several countries where phenacetin sales have been restricted while other analgesics have remained freely available. This has been reported from several countries including the UK (40), Sweden (41), Denmark (42) and Finland (43). These reports were all of fairly short periods of follow-up but the Finns have continued their observations for more than a decade and confirmed the continuing decline (44). In Canada a 50% fall in incidence followed the removal of both phenacetin and paracetamol from mixed analgesics (45). There are some problems in interpreting these studies which have been discussed elsewhere (1) but they do provide substantial support for the thesis that phenacetin plays a special role in human disease.

The counter-argument has been put forward largely from Australia on the basis of two observations: [1] the disease progresses in patients who substitute other analgesics for phenacetin (46). [2] Nationally in Australia the incidence of renal failure from analgesic nephropathy did not fall when sales of phenacetin were restricted but aggressive advertising of other analgesics continued (31).

Progression of renal failure when taking phenacetin-free analgesics

This is a difficult observation to interpret since the disease can progress even if the patients have stopped taking drugs (29). They remain susceptible to the effects of urinary infection, calculus formation and obstruction as well as the spontaneous decline of renal function discussed above. It is universally agreed that patients with analgesic nephropathy should be strongly discouraged from taking further analgesics of any kind. The small minority who have chronic pain unrelieved by other measures should take single analgesics rather than mixtures. However, the role of non-phenacetin containing analgesics in accelerating decline in renal function in this context is not, in my view, sufficiently well documented to weigh heavily in the argument.

Maintained incidence of renal failure from analgesic nephropathy in Australia despite restricted sales of phenacetin

This has remained the most worrying evidence against a predominant role for phenacetin. Analgesic abuse in Australia has been largely confined to two widely advertised brands of powders. Phenacetin was replaced by salicylamide in 1967 in Vincent's Powders and by paracetamol in 1976 in Bex Powders (31). The incidence of renal failure from analgesic nephropathy peaked at 8.4 per million per year in 1980 then declined slowly to 5.5 per million per year in 1988 (47). This is a surprisingly long lag period after the restriction on phenacetin sales. However, more detailed analysis shows that over the period 1977–1988 there was a steep fall in the incidence in the 40–49 age group and a compensating rise in the incidence in the 60–69 age group, peaking in 1984. These data are compatible with the hypothesis that patients with established disease prior to 1977 are continuing to decline into renal failure at progressively older ages (which no longer preclude dialysis and transplant) and are therefore included in Registry figures, while new cases are declining. For confirmation (or refutation) of this theory we await a fuller description of these observations, which is dependent on Australian government funding for the Registry.

Other evidence from Australia supports the importance of phenacetin. McCredie *et al* (48) studied patients with definite and probable papillary necrosis and compared them with normal controls from a population with a high consumption of analgesics by UK standards. Phenacetin-containing analgesics increased the risk of papillary necrosis 17-fold while aspirin alone had no effect.

Paracetamol is the main metabolite of phenacetin and is concentrated in the papilla so many authors, particularly from Australia, have suggested that it is equally nephrotoxic, but with few exceptions there is little support for this in the literature, despite the fact that sales of paracetamol now rival those of aspirin and far exceed those of phenacetin in many countries. Edwards *et al* (49) had the unusual opportunity of studying 18 patients who had taken paracetamol alone in doses up to 30 kg and found no evidence of analgesic nephropathy. Kincaid-Smith (26) mentioned two patients with analgesic nephropathy from consumption of paracetamol alone but gave no further details. Few other cases have been reported from countries such as UK with a high per capita consumption of paracetamol. The international literature, with one exception, supports the consensus view that single analgesics, including paracetamol, rarely, if ever, cause analgesic nephropathy (50).

The exception is Malaysia, where Segasothy and his colleagues (51) have reported 15 patients with papillary necrosis attributed to sole, or predominant, consumption of paracetamol. The reason for this high incidence after consumption of doses varying between 1 and 15 kg in one country is not discernible from the publications. Possible explanations include the hot moist climate of Malaysia, a contaminated brand of paracetamol or an unusual pattern of paracetamol consumption. Speculation must await further published information. It is possible that clinicians in most of the world have failed to detect a drug side effect of this magnitude but this seems unlikely.

Judging the role of paracetamol as a component of analgesic mixtures is more difficult. McCredie and Stewart (52) found no association between paracetamol consumption and papillary necrosis; about half their subjects took paracetamol in mixtures. Two recent large case-control studies (53,54) while confirming a predominant association of renal disease with phenacetin have also shown a weaker association with paracetamol. However, in these studies chronic renal disease included all diagnoses leading to renal impairment (53) or to end stage renal failure (54). I find these studies hard to interpret.

In the German study (54) only a sixth of the patients in renal failure had been diagnosed by their nephrologists as having analgesic nephropathy and the doses of paracetamol consumed were modest—a mean of 770 mg lifelong in those defined as paracetamol takers. This is so far removed from the doses usually taken in analgesic nephropathy as to suggest an artefactual relationship. In the American study (53) 19% of the subjects were classified as having interstitial nephritis but the proportion of these with papillary necrosis or with a clinical diagnosis of analgesic nephropathy was not stated. While it is conceivable that analgesics influence the incidence of many forms of renal disease (including in these series polycystic disease and diabetic nephropathy) it is inherently unlikely and in my view these laborious studies have thrown little light on the role, if any, of paracetamol containing analgesic mixtures.

Aspirin has been accused of a major role in analgesic nephropathy mainly by Australian authors in the period when the incidence of renal failure from analgesic nephropathy was stubbornly refusing to fall after withdrawal of phenacetin but with consumption of aspirin unabated. They have pointed out that it is more nephrotoxic to rats than phenacetin alone, though the two together are synergistic. However, the studies of McCredie and Stewart in New South Wales have lent no support to this view (48,52,55). In the UK Prescott (2), who has contributed so much to the literature on analgesics, has marshalled the case against aspirin in a massive review of the topic. He collected from the literature 82 case reports of patients who had apparently developed analgesic nephropathy after taking aspirin alone. This sounds a formidable case but thirty two of these reports are unpublished cases referred to the Committee on the Safety of Medicines, and many of the remaining 50 have been mentioned only in passing with scanty clinical details. It can be very difficult to obtain a consistent and complete history of analgesic intake over decades and there is therefore a risk of wrongly incriminating a drug in a single case report. One of our recent patients gave me three different estimates of analgesic intake ranging from 2 to 10 kg in three interviews over a fortnight. I have previously commented on one patient with analgesic nephropathy apparently due to consumption of paracetamol alone; when we were on the point of publishing this rare event he remembered seven years' heavy consumption of codeine compound tablets before he started on paracetamol (1).

Consequently I treat with considerable caution the evidence for the nephrotoxicity of aspirin alone.

On the opposite side there is considerable evidence for the lack of nephrotoxicity from aspirin given over many years in therapeutic doses. Groups including the New Zealand Rheumatism Association (56) and Emkey and Mills (57) have studied whole populations of arthritic patients taking aspirin and have failed to find a single case of analgesic nephropathy in more than 1000 patients. At Guy's Hospital (3) and Newcastle (58,59) 46 patients were studied who had taken between 5 and 37 kg of aspirin for arthritis without a single case of analgesic nephropathy being detected. These observations cannot completely exonerate aspirin since analgesic abusers may consume even higher quantities than those used in life long treatment of arthritis. However, they are very reassuring to those using aspirin therapeutically in legitimate doses.

That still leaves open the question whether aspirin plays a part in the causation of analgesic nephropathy when given with other constituents of analgesic mixtures. Epidemiological studies (53,54) give conflicting evidence on this point and suffer from the defects I have discussed above. The Consensus Conference (50) wrote of the pathogenesis of analgesic nephropathy 'Present evidence suggests that acetaminophen causes tissue injury as a result of its conversion to toxic metabolites. By lowering the concentration of glutathione, a substance that protects against tissue injury, aspirin and other salicylates enhance toxicity. These data offer attractive, although yet unproved, explanations for the synergistic effects of phenacetin and aspirin in causing papillary necrosis.' In 1990 it remains an unproved hypothesis but the synergism of these components of analgesic mixtures, at least in rats, is well established. Until the mechanism of this synergism has been elucidated it would seem wise to advise that aspirin should be used alone unless there are compelling reasons for combining it with other agents.

That is already standard medical practice in most countries, but most analgesic nephropathy results from abuse of preparations bought without prescription. Belgium puts a warning on the packet, without much effect so far. Other countries have restricted over-the-counter sales of mixed analgesics, probably with more effect. That benefit is bought at the price of some restriction of personal freedom in self-treatment of minor ailments. Analgesic mixtures were introduced in the belief that giving a small dose of two drugs would give the same benefit, with fewer side effects, as a double dose of a single drug. Now that there is epidemiological evidence (albeit imperfect) that using two drugs may be more nephrotoxic than using one, and a plausible theory to explain why, it seems to me that the onus is on those who wish to market analgesic mixtures to show that they are more efficacious than single drugs or that they produce fewer side effects in other systems (e.g. the gastrointestinal tract) to compensate for the risk of toxicity. In the absence of such evidence, public policy should be to encourage the use of single analgesics.

REFERENCES

(1) Kerr DNS. Renal function after acute or prolonged consumption of aspirin. In: Hallam J, Goldman L and Fryers GR, eds. *Aspirin Symposium 1983*. Royal Society of Medicine International Congress and Symposium Series no. 71. Oxford: Oxford University Press, 1984; 43–8.

(2) Prescott LF. Analgesic nephropathy: A reassessment of the role of phenacetin and other analgesics. *Drugs* 1982; **23**: 75–149.

(3) Burry HC, Dieppe PA, Breshnihan, Brown C. Salicylates and renal function in rheumatoid arthritis. *BMJ* 1976; **2**: 16–17.
(4) Beeley L, Kendall MJ. Effect of aspirin on renal clearance of ^{125}I-diatrizoate. *BMJ* 1971; **1**: 707–8.
(5) Robert M, Fillastre JP, Berger H, Malandain H. Effect of intravenous infusion of acetylsalicylic acid on renal function. *BMJ* 1972; **2**: 466–7.
(6) Burry HC, Dieppa PA. Apparent reduction of endogenous creatinine clearance by salicylate treatment. *BMJ* 1976; **2**: 16–17.
(7) Kimberly RP, Plot PH. Aspirin-induced depression of kidney function. *N Engl J Med* 1977; **296**: 418–24.
(8) Kimberly RP, Bowden RE, Keiser HR, Plotz PH. Reduction of renal function by newer nonsteroidal anti-inflammatory drugs. *Am J Med* 1978; **64**: 804–7.
(9) Kimberly RP, Gill JR, Bowden RE, Keiser HR, Plotz PH. Elevated urinary prostaglandins and the effects of aspirin on renal function in lupus erythematosus. *Ann Intern Med* 1978; **89**: 336–41.
(10) Plotz PH, Kimberly RP. Acute effects of aspirin and acetaminophen on renal function. *Arch Intern Med* 1981; **141**: 343–8.
(11) Arisz L, Donker AJM, Brentjens JRH, van der Hem GK. The effect of indomethacin on proteinuria and kidney function in the nephrotic syndrome. *Acta Med Scand* 1976; **199**: 121–5.
(12) Tweeddale MG, Ogilvie RI. Antagonism of spironolactone-induced natriuresis by aspirin in man. *N Engl J Med* 1973; **289**: 198–200.
(13) Kimberly RP, Sherman RL, Mouradian J, Lockshin MD. Apparent acute renal failure associated with therapeutic aspirin and ibuprofen administration. *Arthritis Rheum* 1979; **22**: 281–5.
(14) Grunefield J-P, Kleinknecht D, Droz D. Acute interstitial nephritis. In: Schrier RW and Gottschalk CW eds. *Diseases of the kidney*. 4th Ed. Boston: Little Brown 1988; 1461–87.
(15) Campbell EJM, Maclaurin RE. Acute renal failure in salicylate poisoning. *BMJ* 1958; **1**: 503–5.
(16) Chapman BJ, Proudfoot AT. Adult salicylate poisoning: deaths and outcome in patients with high plasma salicylate concentrations. *Quart J Med* 1989; **72**: 699–707.
(17) Dreyer NA. Analgesic-associated nephropathy: aetiology or tautology? In: Wood C, ed. *Analgesics and renal disease: who is at risk?* Royal Society of Medicine International Congress and Symposium Series no. 96. London: Royal Society of Medicine 1985; 19–24.
(18) Elseviers MM, De Broe ME. Is analgesic nephropathy still a problem in Belgium? *Nephrol Dial Transplant 1988;* **2**: 143–9.
(19) Bennett WM, De Broe ME. Analgesic nephropathy—a preventable renal disease. *N Engl J Med* 1989; **320**: 1118–23.
(20) Kerr DNS. Clinical and pathological definition of analgesic-associate nephropathy. In: Wood C, ed. *Analgesics and renal disease: who is at risk?* Royal Society of Medicine International Congress and Symposium Series no. 96. London: Royal Society of Medicine 1985; 1–17.
(21) Winearls CG, Kerr DNS. Renal disorders. In: Davies DM, ed. *Textbook of adverse drug reactions*. 3rd Ed. Oxford: Oxford University Press, 1985; 291–334.
(22) Cassidy MJD, Kerr DNS. Renal disorders. In: Davies DM, ed. *Textbook of adverse drug reactions*. 4th Ed. Oxford: Oxford University Press, 1990. In press.
(23) Bell D, Kerr DNS, Swinney J, Yeates WK. Analgesic nephropathy. Clinical course after withdrawal of phenacetin. *BMJ* 1990; **3**: 378–82.
(24) Murray RM, Lawson DH, Linton AL. Analgesic nephropathy: clinical syndrome and prognosis. *BMJ* 1971; **1**: 479–82.
(25) Gàult MH. The clinical course of patients with analgesic nephropathy. *Can Med Assoc J* 1975; **113**: 204–7.
(26) Kincaid-Smith P. Nephrology Forum: analgesic abuse and the kidney. *Kidney Int* 1980; **17**: 250–60.
(27) Burgin M, Schmidt M, Reutter F. Fokal-segmentale Glomerulosklerose bei Analgetika-Naphropathie. *Schweiz Med Wochenschr* 1984; **114**: 1118–23.

(28) Cove-Smith JR. Analgesic-associated kidney disease. *JAMA* 1984; **251**: 3123–5.
(29) Schwarz A, Kunzendorf U, Keller F, Offermann G. Progression of renal failure in analgesic-associated nephropathy. *Nephron* 1989; **53**: 244–9.
(30) Helber A, Wambach G, Bottcher W, Weller P, Schmidt R. Hypercholesterolaemia and hypertriglyceridaemia in patients with analgesic nephropathy. *Nephron* 1980; **26**: 111–5.
(31) Nanra RS, Stuart-Taylor J, de Leon AH, White KH. Analgesic nephropathy: etiology, clinical syndrome, and clinicopathologic correlation in Australia. *Kidney Int* 1978; **13**: 79–92.
(32) Mihatsch MJ, Kernen R, Zollinger HU. Phenacetinabuses VI; eine autopsiestatistik under besonderer Berucksichtignung extrarenaler Befunde. *Schweiz Med Wochenschr* 1982; **112**: 1383–80.
(33) Mora Palma FJ, Ellis HA, Cook DB, *et al.* Osteomalacia in patients with chronic renal failure before dialysis or transplantation. *Quart J Med* 1983; **52**: 332–48.
(34) Fassett RG, Lien JWK, McClure J, Mathew TH. Bone disease in analgesic nephropathy. *Clinc Nephrol* 1982; **18**: 273–9.
(35) Weber M, Braun B, Kohler H. Ultrasonic findings in analgesic nephropathy. *Proc Eur Dial Transpl Assoc* 1983; **20**: 669–84.
(36) Weber M, Braun B, Kohler H. Ultrasonic findings in analgesic nephropathy. *Nephron* 1985; **39**: 216–222.
(37) Jacobs LA, Morris JG. Renal papillary necrosis and the abuse of phenacetin. *Med J Australia* 1962; **2**: 531–8.
(38) Cove-Smith JR. Analgesic nephropathy in the United Kingdom: incidence, clinical features and pathogenesis. *J Clin Pathol* 1981; **34**: 1255–60.
(39) Mihatsch MJ, Hofer HO, Gudat F, *et al.* Capillary sclerosis of the urinary tract and analgesic nephropathy. *Clin Nephrol* 1983; **20**: 285–301.
(40) Murray RM. Analgesic nephropathy: removal of phenacetin from prioretary analgesics. *BMJ* 1972; **4**: 131–2.
(41) Nordenfelt O. Deaths from renal failure in abusers of phenacetin-containing drugs. *Acta Med Scand* 1972; **191**: 11–16.
(42) Mabeck CE, Wichman B. Mortality from chronic interstitial nephritis and phenacetin consumption in Denmark. *Acta Med Scand* 1979; **205**: 599–601.
(43) Kasanen A. The effect of the restriction of the sale of phenacetin on the incidence of papillary necrosis established at autopsy. *Ann Clin Res* 1973; **5**: 369–74.
(44) Sillanpaa M, Kasanen A, Elonen A. Changes of panorama in renal disease mortality in Finland after phenacetin restriction. *Acta Med Scand* 1982; **212**: 313–7.
(45) Korcok M. Medical News: Analgesic nephropathy dips in Canada after mixture ban. *JAMA* 1981; **246**: 2008.
(46) Kincaid-Smith P, Nanra RS, Fairley KF. Analgesic nephropathy: a recoverable form of chronic renal failure. In: Kincaid-Smith P, Fairley KF, eds. *Renal infection and renal scarring*. Melbourne: Mercedes 1971; 385–400.
(47) Disney APS, ed. *Twelfth Report of the Australian and New Zealand Combined Dialysis and Transplant Registry*. Queen Elizabeth Hospital, Woodville, South Australia 1989.
(48) McCredie M, Stewart JH, Mahony JF. Is phenacetin responsible for analgesic nephropathy in New South Wales? *Clin Nephrol* 1982; **17**: 134–40.
(49) Edwards OM, Edwards P, Huskisson EC, Taylor RT. Paracetamol and renal damage. *BMJ* 1971; **2**: 87–9.
(50) Consensus conference. Analgesic-associated kidney disease. *JAMA* 1984; **251**: 3123–5.
(51) Segasothy M, Suleiman AB, Puvaneswary M, Rohana A. Paracetamol: a cause for analgesic nephropathy and end-stage renal disease. *Nephron* 1988; **50**: 50–4.
(52) McCredie M, Stewart JH. Does paracetamol cause urothelial cancer or papillary necrosis? *Nephron* 1988; **49**: 296–300.
(53) Sandler DP, Smith JC, Weinberg CR, *et al.* Analgesic use and chronic renal disease. *N Engl J Med* 1989; **320**: 1238–43.
(54) Pommer W, Brondr E, Greiser E, *et al.* Regular analgesic intake and the risk of end-stage renal failure. *Am J Nephrol* 1989; **9**: 403–12.

(55) McCredie M, Stewart JH, Mathew TH, Disney APS, Ford JM. The effect of withdrawal of phenacetin-containing analgesics and the incidence of kidney and urothelial cancer and renal failure. *Clin Nephrol* 1989; **31**: 35–9.
(56) New Zealand Rheumatism Association Study. Aspirin and the kidney. *BMJ* 1974; **1**: 593–6.
(57) Emkey RD, Mills JA. Aspirin and analgesic nephropathy still a problem in Belgium? *Nephrol Dial Transpl* 1988; **2**: 143–9.
(58) Mackon AF, Craft AW, Thompson M, Kerr DNS. Aspirin and analgesic nephropathy. *BMJ* 1974; **1**: 597–600.
(59) Akyol SM, Thompson M, Kerr DNS. Renal function after prolonged consumption of aspirin. *BMJ* 1982; **284**: 631–2.

Aspirin in the treatment of juvenile arthritis

John Baum

School of Medicine and Dentistry, University of Rochester, New York, USA

INTRODUCTION

I would like to claim that rheumatologists have primacy in the use of aspirin in human disease treatment because, of course, aspirin was first used for arthritis. Even salicylate goes back to the 1890s for treatment of children with arthritis. I must also point out that many of the diseases which we deal with in juvenile age group (up to 16 years) are diseases which require, not simply analgesics, but anti-inflammatory medication.

In the differential diagnosis of juvenile arthritis (JA) we deal with a number of other types of diseases: systemic lupus erythematosus, dermatomyositis, polyarteritis, Kawasaki's disease. The latter, for example, is a disease in which it is well known that arthritis is one of the major drugs used. In the prevention of the coronary aneurysms it, together with IV γ-globulin, even provided better results than with steroids (1). Rheumatic fever, which unfortunately has been having a minor resurgence in the USA, is another disease which we know has responded very well over the years to aspirin therapy. It is quite interesting that, of all the juvenile diseases, I see the reddest joints appear to be in those with rheumatic fever.

There are other diseases in which we do not use aspirin except for analgesia, and these are the arthritides due to infection. Lyme Disease for instance has become a major problem on the East coast of the USA and, in Philadelphia it has become a more important cause of admission to the Children's Hospital than even juvenile arthritis.

HYPERMOBILITY SYNDROME

I would like to discuss non-joint problems where we have used aspirin. Hypermobility syndrome is typical and is a condition more commonly present than recognized.

This is a syndrome which can be easily diagnosed, and which was first identified in England. We found it in about 6% of our population of children referred to an arthritis clinic because they had what appeared to be a joint problem, but which could not be identified by their physician (2). We believe that its frequency in the population is, therefore, higher. The characteristics are: the affected knee joints

Aspirin—towards 2000, edited by G. R. Fryers, 1990; Royal Society of Medicine Services International Congress and Symposium Series No. 168, published by Royal Society of Medicine Services Limited.

go back to greater than 10°, the fingers can be bent back parallel to the forearm, the thumb can be brought down to touch the forearm: hyperextension to 10° or more at the elbow, and being able to bend over and put the palms flat on the ground.

This condition is not a minor problem; we find it in a good number of the population and aspirin seems to provide the best therapy. The hypermobility syndrome is more common in females, and has been described as showing three or more hypermobile joints. We now feel that if a child has one hypermobile joint, which would be a larger percentage of the population, and they do something which stresses that joint and then suffer pain because of it, then this would also be due to hypermobility, and could be called the hypermobility syndrome. I would like to point out that reassurance and symptomatic treatment with aspirin provides the best therapy.

There is a condition which is sometimes known as 'growing pains'. Paediatricians talk about it and a Danish physician sought to show that it ran in families (3). I am beginning to feel that what has been called growing pains by many physicians may actually be the hypermobility syndrome. Growing pains appear at night, and it seems that children with hypermobility syndrome have a lot of their symptoms at night, especially after they have been very active during the day. We believe that the joint which is hypermobile suffers some stress and results in pain later on. We have been very successful in using enteric coated aspirin at bedtime, because the major effect of this dosage appears during the night. We have seen children who were waking nightly, who, after aspirin, were sleeping throughout the night.

JUVENILE ARTHRITIS

Juvenile arthritis has proved easier to treat when one can subdivide what used to be called juvenile rheumatoid arthritis into several different conditions. For example, there is a difference between those who have rheumatoid factor present and those who do not. The term juvenile rheumatoid arthritis should be reserved for those in whom rheumatoid factor is part of the disease.

Aspirin is widely used to treat these conditions. In several series where aspirin has been tested against other non-steroidal anti-inflammatory drugs (NSAIDs), both in adults and children, one of the major causes for aspirin being discontinued, or for poor patient compliance, was gastro-intestinal irritation. However, studies with enteric coated aspirin have shown a number of problems with aspirin are diminished and gastric haemorrhage and ulceration no longer appeared as a major problem (4). In fact, for safety's sake and because, interestingly enough, an enteric coated tablet is easier to swallow because it has a very smooth coating, most of the children that I treat with aspirin are given the enteric coated variety. The non-aspirin salicylates are also used to some extent.

In the USA at present, the only other NSAIDs used which have been approved by the Federal Drug Administration are tolmetin and naproxen. Naproxen has an advantage in young children because it comes in a liquid preparation, so that children between the ages of one and three years who cannot or do not wish to swallow tablets are able to accept this treatment. We do use analgesics, and I use most that are available including paracetamol and codeine. We also use corticosteroids in both the oral form and intra-articularly.

There are also long-acting agents or disease modifying agents. However, we have done some collaborative studies with the Russians, finding that hydroxychloroquine and D-penicillamine were not better than placebo when tested in a population of children with arthritis (5). Auranofin (oral gold), seems to be better than these drugs. Sulfasalazine is being used and is being tested, as is methotrexate and I think that these drugs will be shown to be effective.

Being able to divide arthritis in children into different categories made therapy a little more rational and a little better to use. We do use NSAIDs in all the categories; the analgesics I add when I have reached what I consider to be a maximum dose of NSAID. The advantage of aspirin still remains that, if you give a certain dose and see no effect, you still get a salicylate level. If the salicylate level is low you know you can increase the dose: if it is high you know you have reached the maximum amount you can give. This is still an advantage which is not shared by any of the other NSAIDs and I think is particularly important when treating children.

Corticosteroids are used, but there is no well-defined point when to use them as there is to some degree with adults. Intra-articular corticosteroids are sometimes useful when a child has one or two joints which are particularly troublesome. Again, this is the same type of therapy we use in adult rheumatoid arthritis.

The long-acting agents are used mostly in the polyarticular type. I do not use them in the pauciarticular disease (defined as 5 or fewer joints, mostly large joints of the lower extremities) except sometimes for young boys with HLA-B27 disease, where we are starting to use sulfasalazine. In pauciarticular disease we use mostly NSAIDs.

The systemic type of juvenile arthritis is called Still's disease after George Frederick Still, the English paediatrician who first described it in 1897. This type is difficult to treat; we try NSAIDs, and if aspirin does not work we try some of the others where we can raise the dosage to extremely high levels. I sometimes use 2–3 times the recommended dose. If they do not work, we go on to corticosteroids, and now with some we are using methotrexate. These children have high spiking fevers, high white counts, high erythrocyte sedimentation rates, a rash, hepatosplenomegaly and lymphadenopathy. One would expect the cause to be a virus, but these children have been cultured from every orifice and nothing that has ever been grown is incriminating. We are beginning to look more closely at genetics in all these conditions.

EFFECTS OF ASPIRIN

In 1977 the Pediatric Rheumatology Collaborative Study Group in the USA undertook a study comparing aspirin and tolmetin. The point was: what does aspirin do? We finally knew just where aspirin was most helpful (6): it significantly reduced morning stiffness, it reduced the number of painful joints, it did not seem to have a major effect on swollen or active joints, it did improve joints with limited motion. Morning stiffness is a very good indicator of inflammatory activity and aspirin can work on swollen joints rather rapidly.

Serum glutamic oxalo-acetic transaminase (ALT) and serum glutamic pyruvic transaminase (AST), which become elevated with initial aspirin therapy, showed no significant changes in children after three months of aspirin. In this collaborative study we (6) examined the AST and ALT in children in a double-blind fashion. Children who had been on aspirin before the study and then were studied double-blind, showed the originally elevated levels of these enzymes then fell to within the normal range with tolectin. When they were in the aspirin portion, the levels initially rose a little, possibly because they were now taking aspirin on a more regular basis, then started to fall. Another interesting point is that the enzymes fell to nearly, but not quite, normal levels. Even if children have abnormal levels of these enzymes they will tend to fall after an initial peak.

In these papers the results were pooled to see why various drugs had to be discontinued. For example, there were cases of diminished hearing with aspirin but there was no alopecia with aspirin that we saw with some of the other NSAIDs. Mouth ulcers were not reported in any of our children with aspirin. Change in personality is not well-known but was reported with aspirin and may be related to salicylism.

Aspirin therapy varies from country to country; every country has its own way of giving medication, and I compared what they did in USSR with what was done in the USA. In the Soviet Union they gave a short course of aspirin before going on to other drugs, while in the USA we were more conscious of cost perhaps, and maintained aspirin for longer periods of time (7).

RESPONSE TIME

A very important analysis (8) looked at the time course of response to a number of NSAIDs. No matter what type of juvenile arthritis it was, the response continued to go up slowly, but it took 12 weeks before *all* those who eventually responded did so. All of these drugs take time for a significant response to appear. For example, if we take those children whom we considered to have a favourable response after three months and looked at the drugs, in days before response appears, the mean for aspirin was 30 days, shorter than with the other drugs. The median for aspirin was 18 days, (minimum 13 days, maximum 107 days). Thus when I deal with a parent I say: 'I am going to give this child aspirin. You may not see an effect for weeks, but do not worry because we may have to give it for three weeks to a month and maybe longer before we know whether or not it actually will work, although some chldren respond more quickly.'

By week 8, the percentage of the responders already responding was still only 80%. These drugs may work quickly, but to achieve maximal response in a patient, you must give it for at least 12 weeks. I usually give eight weeks as my treatment, aiming for the 80% level and say: 'If it does not work in two months we will probably go on to another drug and see how that works, but you have to be patient because it may take time for the drug to work.' Among the non-responders, a quarter responded right up to eight weeks but by 12 weeks there was no further response in the others.

REYE'S SYNDROME

I am a clinician and I have to be aware of Reye's syndrome, as well as explaining it to parents. The trouble is that salicylism and Reye's syndrome are very similar except for serum amino acids. The glutamine, alanine and lysine levels are said to be elevated, but this is not universally believed. I believe that liver biopsy is needed to determine what is going on. Even a viral illness could be present as the problem, when you are dealing with chronic salicylism. I know of cases of Reye's syndrome in juvenile arthritis, in which the levels of serum salicylate appeared to be well in the range of what I would call salicylism!

I deal in the United States with an increasingly litigious society. We pay a large amount of money for malpractice insurance and Reye's syndrome is always in the background of aspirin therapy. I handle it by being honest with the patients. I tell the mothers that there is an entity they have perhaps read about, known as Reye's syndrome which has been linked in some studies to aspirin. I follow the advice to tell the parent that, if there should be a viral epidemic, principally of influenza or chicken pox, they are to stop the aspirin and let the physician know about it. I give the aspirin and say it is a good and cheap drug which should work in the arthritis but, if it does not, we have other drugs. If there is any question of influenza about, if the child looks as though they are getting any of the viral syndromes, they are to stop the aspirin and let me know. I will also be careful to follow the child with serum salicylate levels, and if a child does start vomiting or does have gastric upset I tell the mother that I want to see that child right away and we will determine the salicylate level and check that child out with the other tests that have been described.

I have not seen a case of Reye's syndrome in 30 years of treating children with juvenile arthritis and similar conditions. But, since the odds against my ever seeing it are high, even if a case were to develop I would continue to use aspirin as well as the other NSAIDs. Vigilance is really the best defence against any unusual or untoward symptoms, plus the very good tool of being able to measure salicylate level, so that if chronic salicylism is the cause of the child's symptoms we can pick it up immediately.

REFERENCES

(1) Hicks R. Kawasaki's diseases. *XVIIth Con ILAR Congress of Rheumatology* Rio de Janiero, 21 September 1989.

(2) Biro MD, Gewanter HL, Baum J. The hypermobility syndrome. *Pediatrics* 1983; **71**: 701–6.

(3) Oster J. Growing pains. *Danish Med Bull* 1972; **19**: 72–9.

(4) Lanza FL, Rach MF, Wagner GS, Balm TK. Reduction in gastric mucosal hemorrhage and ulceration with chronic high-level dosing of enteric-coated aspirin granules two and four times a day. *Dig Dis Sci* 1985; **30**: 509–12.

(5) Brewer EJ Jr, Giannini EH, Kuzmina N, Alekseer L. Penicilliumine and hydroxychloroquine in the treatment of severe juvenile rheumatoid arthritis. *N Engl J Med* 1986; **314**: 1269–76.

(6) Levinson JE, Baum J, Brewer EJ Jr, Fink C, Hanson V, Schaller J. Comparison of tolmetin sodium and aspirin in the treatment juvenile rheumatoid arthritis. *J Pediatr* 1977; **91**: 799–804.

(7) Baum J, Alekseer LS, Brewer EJ Jr, Dolgopolova AV, Mudhokar G, Patel K. Juvenile rheumatoid arthritis: a comparison of patients from the USSR and USA. *Arthritis Rheum* 1980; **23**: 977–84.

(8) Lovell DJ, Giannini EH, Brewer EJ Jr. Time course of response to non-steroidal antiinflammatory drugs in juvenile rheumatoid arthritis. *Arthritis Rheum* 1984; **27**: 1433–7.

DISCUSSION

Dr Graham: If a GP diagnoses hypermobility syndrome, is it reasonable to go on treating it in general practice and, if aspirin is contraindicated, what should he use?

Professor Baum: It can be treated with any analgesic agent, though the children who wake up at night seem to do better with enteric coated aspirin. That is a trick because you get a later dissolution of the tablet and so, at the time that the child is usually having the symptoms, you get the major effect. However, they will respond to any analgesic, and they respond best to a definition of the disease, because usually, by the time they see me in a paediatric arthritis clinic, the parents have been to a number of doctors. I had a parent recently who had been to five or six different physicians of all types because of the continued pain. The child was extremely hypermobile and, what is fascinating about this condition, it had not been recognized. I have had a family come in where the child was very hypermobile and I asked the mother: 'Did you know your child could do these things?' and I asked the child to put her leg around her neck. She said: 'No, I never knew that.' I said: 'Do you have any other children. Are any of them like this?' She said: 'I don't know, but they are outside.' I brought them in and both were as hypermobile as the child who had every one of the five features present. So it is something that people can live with and not be recognized. From our population survey we believe that features of it are present in a large number of individuals.

Does aspirin prevent cataracts?

John Harding

Nuffield Laboratory of Ophthalmology, Oxford, UK

INTRODUCTION

The lens is contained within a collagenous capsule, a basement membrane-like structure, and inside the front of the capsule there is a single layer of epithelial cells which divide, move to the equator, and elongate into the long fibre cells that fill most of the lens. During this elongation process they lose their nuclei. The cells build up in this way like an onion, with the new cells on the outside of the old cells, so in the centre of the lens there are cells that were there before birth, and there is no protein turnover, no synthesis detectable in this part of the lens, which contains the oldest proteins in the body.

It is not surprising that, with age, these proteins sustain a certain amount of damage, which accumulates because the proteins are not renewed, as they are in most other tissues. If the damage becomes excessive the lens becomes opaque and milky and light no longer passes through the lens to the retina. An opaque lens is a cataract.

There are many different pathways to cataract but we are trying to find common pathways in different types with different risk factors, and one common pathway to cataract is through chemical modification of the lens proteins. If we take, for example, a major risk factor for cataract in Western countries, diabetes, it is associated with high glucose levels and high levels of glucose 6-phosphate and other sugar metabolites, and the glucose can react with proteins. When it reacts with proteins it causes them to unfold, which we have been able to demonstrate *in vitro*, and that can lead on to aggregation and cataract.

But, just as glucose can react with proteins, some of the steroids that are associated with cataract react with proteins: cyanate, derived from urea that is elevated in renal failure, can react with proteins and they all do much the same thing. They all react with amino groups, they all change the charges on the surface of the proteins, and unfold them.

ASPIRIN AND CATARACT

Some years ago Cotlier (1) produced evidence that aspirin protected against cataract in rheumatoid arthritis and diabetes patients. At that time we were working on the chemical modification of protein and this protection seemed

Aspirin—towards 2000, edited by G. R. Fryers, 1990; Royal Society of Medicine Services International Congress and Symposium Series No. 168, published by Royal Society of Medicine Services Limited.

unlikely because I knew that aspirin acetylated proteins and I had come to feel that anything which chemically modified proteins was very bad for the lens. But we found that aspirin could prevent some of these chemical modifications, by cyanate or by sugars. Salicylate does not work in this system, nor does salicylate prevent the original reaction of cyanate with the proteins (2).

We looked at the non-enzymic glycosylation reaction, and found it also associated with cataract. We get very similar results with cyanate and with sugars, with glucose 6-phosphate and with glucosamine, both of which are increased in diabetes (3,4). So aspirin certainly appears to have some protective effects for the lens *in vitro*.

OXFORD CATARACT STUDY

Before we had these results we had started a case-controlled study of cataract in Oxford which was designed to look for risk factors for cataract. It was not looking for protective effects as we were not aware that there were any. In that study, carried out by interview, there were 300 cases from the Oxford Eye Hospital, cataract patients at the time of cataract surgery so that they had real visually impairing cataract, and 609 controls, some hospital-derived and some from the community. Subjects were aged 50–79 years and the controls were age and sex matched to the cases so the mean age was about 70 years.

They were asked for a full medical history, but there was also a question about drugs that simply asked what drugs they had taken regularly for at least four months at some time in their life. In answer to that it was seen that 7.2% of the controls, and 5% of the cases reported having taken aspirin regularly for at least four months at some time in their life. Although there seems to be an excess in controls, and of course with a risk factor you find an excess in the cases, here the aspirin does appear to be tending towards a protective effect. This result was not significant. However, we noticed that, not just aspirin, but paracetamol, ibuprofen and similar drugs all tended towards a protective effect. When the drugs were pooled, increasing the numbers, the aspirin-like analgesics were reported by 30% of the controls but only 17% of the cases. Using the X^2 test, this is highly significant, with a relative risk of about 0.47, so according to this study, consumption of these drugs regularly for at least four months is associated with an approximate halving of the risk of cataract (5).

Of course, at the end of this study, although we were happy to confirm Professor Cotlier's results with aspirin, and we were also happy to find a result for the other drugs, we had the problem of what dose of these drugs might be useful. If someone was going to start a clinical trial, and I urged people to do so, they wanted to know how much of the drug they should give to the patients and we could not give an answer because of the nature of the question. So we set up a second case-controlled study with a fairly similar design, with 423 cases, 608 controls age and sex matched, and similar questions about medical history.

Diabetes is well known as a risk factor for cataract, and in this second study we found it to be reported by 3.6% of the controls and about 14% of the cases. The difference is highly significant and the relative risk is about four (6), that is, diabetes increases the risk of cataract about four-fold in this age group.

More important, we were able to confirm the protective effect of aspirin-like analgesics. We had on the questionnaire the same question as in the first study about regular consumption of drugs for more than four months, and found a similar result. However, we had extra questions about dose, what analgesic people had taken, what dose level, when they started and when they stopped. Here, taking either aspirin, paracetamol or ibuprofen at any dose level we had 45% of controls reporting and only 30% of cases, and the difference was highly significant; a relative risk of about 0.5 with a very narrow confidence interval (7). The whole group of drugs is associated with a very highly significant protective effect. The people who reported aspirin included 14.5% controls and 7.6% cases, the difference again being highly significant, and the relative risk again about 0.5.

It could be argued that the effect of aspirin was only because people taking aspirin will at some time have taken paracetamol or ibuprofen and maybe one of those drugs has the real effect. It is not easy to disentangle these possibilities, but there are programs now that will do so and we have used a linear modelling program called GLIM and by two different types of analysis were able to show that any dose of these drugs was associated with an independent protective effect, so aspirin, independently of any consumption of paracetamol or ibuprofen, was associated with a protective effect.

Looking at the doses more carefully we divided the subjects into quartiles according to their aspirin consumption, and even those patients in the lowest quartile of aspirin consumption appeared to be protected against cataract. There was again a greater proportion of controls than cases; the difference is significant. The numbers are smaller now so the level of significance is not as good ($p=0.012$), and again there is a low relative risk with a slightly wider confidence interval but still significantly below 1.

The upper end of the lowest quartile is in fact a total remembered consumption of about 150 g aspirin—450 tablets. So this rather low total dose of aspirin is associated with a protective effect.

Of course, these epidemiological studies do not on their own demonstrate whether a risk factor is a causal factor, nor whether a protective factor is really itself directly protective, or whether the consumption of the drug may be associated with something else that could be protective. The most obvious thing would be that the condition for which the drug is taken may be protective. The people who took aspirin gave many reasons, some of which have not been mentioned even at this conference, such as helping them to sleep, giving them confidence, but more than anything else people mentioned arthritis. About 46% of the controls and 44% of cases reported arthritis, a very similar proportion, and clearly arthritis is not itself a protective factor and therefore cannot be the cause of the aspirin and similar drugs appearing as a protective factor. In fact, when we look at our data and the background of what has been done on aspirin in laboratories, as well as other studies, then most of the accepted criteria of a causal relationship are satisfied. It does appear to me that aspirin and the other drugs protect against cataract in man. However, the next step should be for a properly conducted clinical trial of aspirin, paracetamol or ibuprofen to test this notion.

PROTECTIVE MECHANISM

Our main problem now is to ask the question: what is the mechanism for this? The *in vitro* studies were easily explained by acetylation, and Cotlier will discuss that more fully. Acetylation protects the lens proteins against non-enzymic modification, not only glycosylation but carbamylation and other reactions, but of course you cannot explain the action of ibuprofen in the same way because it cannot acetylate proteins. Maybe we do not need to explain the effect of all the drugs in the same way. They may act in different ways but the results are very similar for each one. Aspirin and ibuprofen are both known to lower blood glucose, to stimulate insulin production. Professor Linner from Sweden has suggested (personal communication) that they might improve blood flow to the eye; there are other possibilities including decreasing the formation of malondialdehyde, a side product from thromboxane synthesis which might get round to the lens, and certainly what is normally measured as malondialdehyde has been found in the lens. We are not sure what the mechanism is, which makes it more difficult to establish a causal relationship, but I think the evidence points in that direction.

REFERENCES

(1) Cotlier E, Sharma YG, Niven T, Brescia M. Distribution of salicylate in lens and intraocular fluids and its effect on cataract formation. *Am J Med* 1983; **74**: 83–90.
(2) Crompton M, Rixon KC, Harding JJ. Aspirin prevents carbamylation of soluble lens proteins and prevents cyanate-induced phase separation opacities *in vitro*: A possible mechanism by which aspirin could prevent cataract. *Exp Eye Res* 1985; **40**: 297–311.
(3) Huby R, Harding JJ. Non-enzymic glycosylation (glycation) of lens proteins by galactose and protection by aspirin and reduced glutathione. *Exp Eye Res* 1988; **47**: 53–9.
(4) Ajiboye R, Harding JJ. The non-enzymic glycosylation of bovine lens proteins by glucosamine and its inhibition by aspirin, ibuprofen and glutathione. *Exp Eye Res* 1989; **49**: 31–41.
(5) Harding JJ, van Heyningen R. Drugs, including alcohol, that act as risk factors for cataract, and possible protection against cataract by aspirin-like analgesics and cyclopenthiazide. *Br J Ophthalmol* 1988; **72**: 809–14.
(6) Harding JJ, Harding RS, Egerton M. Risk factors for cataract in Oxfordshire: diabetes, peripheral neuropathy, myopia, glaucoma and diarrhoea. *Acta Ophthalmol* 1989 (in press).
(7) Harding JJ, Egerton M, Harding RS. Protection against cataract by aspirin, paracetamol and ibuprofen. *Acta Ophthalmol* 1989 (in press).

Acetylation of lens crystallins and prevention of diabetic and steroid cataracts

Edward Cotlier

Department of Ophthalmology, King Saud University, Riyadh, Saudi Arabia

INTRODUCTION

Cataract is an opacity or group of opacities in the crystalline lens and it is a very important cause of blindness and decreased vision around the world. We need the lens in the eye in order to see clearly, in the same way as a photographic camera needs a clear lens to get a good picture. If there is opacity in the lens, or the lens is partially cloudy, then visual acuity decreases markedly and we cannot see properly.

Eight years ago I reported for the first time (1,2) that patients who had taken aspirin for long periods of time had a decreased prevalence of cataract. This was a group of patients with rheumatoid arthritis, to which I then added a series of patients with osteoarthritis. The series was collected from patients in the New Haven area, all of whom had been admitted to the Yale University School of Medicine for arthritis, and their consumption of aspirin had been recorded by three different observers. In addition to questioning the patient, the senior physician, the physician in charge and the junior resident had recorded the intake of aspirin and they had followed this through several years so it was well-documented evidence of how much aspirin they had taken and for how long. Using the criterion of $\leqslant$20/30 vision, we found that the patients who had taken aspirin had a low prevalence of cataract, 14%. Those who did not take aspirin had 43% and this was very significant. Also, a group of diabetic patients with rheumatoid arthritis who had taken aspirin had 20% prevalence of cataracts, compared to 78% among those who had not taken aspirin. I was impressed from the very beginning by this significant difference between these groups of patients, particularly when the osteoarthritis group showed similar effects.

The questions raised at the time were: how does aspirin work on the lens, and what mechanisms could be operative to get this effect? I was at a loss to explain it at the time. At the first meeting of the Aspirin Foundation it was suggested that it might be because aspirin is a good acetylation agent, but I did not then see much difference between aspirin and salicylate, and I suspected the effect of salicylate might be important. In the last five years, with the collaboration of Dr G. Rao, a biochemist who worked with me at Yale but is now at the Emory University School of Medicine, and with Dr Robert Urban, and in collaboration

Aspirin—towards 2000, edited by G. R. Fryers, 1990; Royal Society of Medicine Services International Congress and Symposium Series No. 168, published by Royal Society of Medicine Services Limited.

with a team led by Dr A. Cerami at the Rockefeller Institute, we tried to solve the basic mechanism for aspirin effects on the lens.

DIABETIC CATARACT

In two particular types of cataract, in diabetic and steroid cataracts, how do we explain the aspirin effect? First, diabetic cataract. There are two types, a juvenile type characterized by vacuoles, and by a tremendous amount of swelling in the lens, due to the fact that glucose rushes into the lens, where it is converted into a sugar alcohol known as sorbitol by an enzyme called aldose reductase and then produces a lot of nicotinamide-adenine-dinucleotide phosphate (NADPH) oxidation. This lowers the glutathione in the lens and creates a substantial water and sodium imbalance; the lens becomes swollen like a tissue that cannot maintain its low concentration of water. Insulin treatment more or less reverses this cataract because the swelling of the lens subsides.

There is also an adult-onset diabetic type of cataract and this is more related to senile cataract, in that these are patients who have an anticipation or an earlier presentation of senile cataract. Instead of developing senile cataract at age 65–70 like most people, they begin to develop senile-type cataract at age 45–50 years, so that they are about 10 years earlier in the presentation of their cataract. This is due to the fact that diabetes accelerates the ageing process in the lens. Recognition of this type of cataract is due to the work of Cerami at the Rockefeller Institute (3), and of Harding at Oxford (4,5). The cataract results from glycosylation of crystallins; glucose attaches to the proteins of the lens, the glucose changes the conformation of the protein and then the proteins age very quickly to become opaque.

Glycosylation is a process by which glucose is attached to the amino groups of proteins, in this case the lens, which has amino groups that are available. The lens has more protein than any other tissue in the body; the human adult lens is 50–60% protein; while the animal lens has about 35%, so there is plenty to be glycosylated, far more than haemoglobin, for example. Although the terminals of the proteins are protected, and curiously enough protected by acetyl groups in the normal condition, there are lysine groups in the protein itself which are exposed to glucose and glucose readily attaches to it.

The glycation of the lens crystallins will form high molecular weight aggregates, the proteins become bigger and bigger, sometimes in molecular weights of 10^6; this produces bonds and creates changes in the transparency of the lens.

This was initially demonstrated by experiments at the Rockefeller Institute by Cerami and his group. They devoted a number of years to the problem and found that glycated proteins were opaque, whereas non-glycated proteins or non-glycated crystallins, were clear (3). This process can be developed in the test tube within 3–4 weeks. We, and many others, have been able to reproduce these results, not only with mixed crystallins but also with the individual α, β and γ crystallins, separated on the basis of molecular weight.

ASPIRIN AND DIABETIC CATARACT

We then realized that, as aspirin has acetyl groups available, it could attach the acetyl groups to these amino groups of the crystallins and be protective against glycosylation. Thus, we incubated the crystallins with aspirin to see what happened. The first experiments showed, very importantly, that aspirin can acetylate the crystallins of the lens (6,7). We wanted to know whether the acetyl groups of the aspirin would attach to the crystallins, and does it have a permanent bond to the crystallins of the lens. We took a homogenized preparation of calf and human lenses, centrifuged the crystallins and then put them in columns to separate the various types of crystallin before acetylating each with ^{14}C aspirin that was labelled either in the acetyl group or the carboxyl group. Of course, if something is in the carboxyl group it will not acetylate the proteins and if it is in the acetyl group it will show as radioactivity. We used standard methods for acetylation which have been used for red blood cells and other acetylated proteins, and we published the first report in 1985 (6). This was done with the acetylation of crystallins with cold aspirin in the calf lens, but our more recent work with the human lens (7) showed very similar results.

Basically it means that the acetyl group of aspirin will attach to the individual crystallins and, no matter how much you wash them or dialyse them, the proteins will be acetylated. We then discovered that, not only is the acetylation virtually permanent, but it also protects the crystallins from subsequent chemical modifications (7).

The α crystallins are more readily acetylated than the other two types of crystallin, even more than the γ crystallin, and this behaviour relates to the number of amino groups possessed by the crystallin. The α crystallins have more amino groups, more lysine available, and consequently more can be acetylated, whereas the γ crystallins have less, so less is acetylated. So we found also a good relationship between the type of crystallin and the acetylation process.

When we used the 'cold' aspirin, we measured the amino groups in the aspirin-treated preparations and the controls, showing that aspirin-treated preparations will acetylate the α crystallins more than the β crystallins and more than the γ crystallins, whereas the sulphydryl groups that are not supposed to be acetylated are not affected by aspirin. I would say that from the basic science viewpoint everything is established. It is obvious that the acetylation takes place where it is supposed to, in the crystallins that have the high content of amino groups.

When we acetylated the crystallins with aspirin and then exposed them to radioactive glucose we were able to block the glycosylation process in the aspirin-treated crystallins, even in the γ crystallins (7) We are satisfied that we have determined a basic mechanism to explain why aspirin has an effect in protecting against this type of diabetic cataract.

Abrahams' group in Georgia, USA, found that in animals the glycosylation process takes place rather slowly, because the diabetic cataract develops slowly, and also there is glycation of 14–15% of the proteins (8). Abrahams and his group were able to demonstrate that glycation takes place in the diabetic rat (8). If aspirin is added to a protein which is being glycated *in vitro*, it will block the amount of glycated protein and, in a few days, you can also decrease the formation of high molecular weight aggregates in the aspirin-treated as compared to the non-aspirin treated. This provides independent confirmation that, at least in experimental animals, aspirin works by preventing glycation in the lens.

In rats that are receiving aspirin, as compared to those not receiving aspirin, the high molecular weight aggregates of the crystallins are also markedly decreased, and the severity of the cataract in the experimental animals is also markedly decreased in the aspirin-treated animals (2). We have already undertaken some experiments with galactosaemia which were published in the *American Journal of Medicine Aspirin Symposium* (2), showing that aspirin or salicylate causes the formation of cataracts in galactosaemic animals to decrease. Again, this is an indication that there is good basic science that can be reproduced, not only *in vitro* but also in the experimental animal. The acute cataract in animals takes place in a very short period of time and it is similar to the juvenile cataract in humans, in that there are vacuoles and hydration in the lens.

We wondered whether aspirin has any effect on inhibition of the formation of sorbitol, and perhaps protecting against the oxidation of NADPH in the lens, for this is a very important mechanism for the juvenile form of cataract. We had found that aldose reductase, which converts glucose to sorbitol, can be inhibited by aspirin, and by salicylate as well as by other agents. We think this reaction is important inasmuch as it uses a lot of NADPH and the lens deteriorates rapidly when it does not have sufficient NADPH. Our initial results, presented at the previous Aspirin Symposium (2), were confirmed independently by a group using nuclear magnetic resonance spectroscopy to demonstrate that salicylic acid and acetylsalicylic acid are inhibitors of the aldose reductase reaction, so protecting against the utilization of NADPH (9).

It is important to note that the concentrations of aspirin taken by humans are much higher than other compounds tested, such as indomethacin, sulindac and tolrestat, so these compounds inhibit at lower concentrations. Aspirin, a drug administered in high concentrations, is able to provide an antioxidant effect that is exerted at the level of the NADPH. And when we measure the NADPH oxidation by this system, using a substrate glyceraldehyde, we find that sulindac, indomethacin, salicylate, oxyphenbutazone are very good inhibitors of this reaction (2).

STEROID CATARACTS

Steroids have keto carbohydrate-like groups which can also bind to the lens proteins and produce cataract. These corticosteroid cataracts result from high doses of topical or systemic steroids in patients who have rheumatoid arthritis, osteoarthritis, or a number of other conditions, such as transplant surgery. Cerami's group at the Rockefeller Institute believed that they had a similar mechanism by which steroids can produce cataracts, postulating that prednisone attaches to the lysine amino groups, produces an adduct and undergoes a rearrangement. This adduct, they suggested, is the reason why the crystallins are modified and the cataract develops (3,10,11). The hypothesis was proven very easily by incubating either crystallins with steroids, prednisone, or by injecting prednisone into the eye and producing conformational changes in the crystallins. There is then aggregation with formation of disulphide groups and when the aggregates occur, the proteins become opaque and the lens loses its transparency (3,10).

Most interestingly, when we incubated crystallins with prednisone, we could block the opacification of the crystallins by aspirin over a period of 25–30 days (11). Once again a similar mechanism has been helped by understanding that acetylation of crystallins has a protective effect on protein aggregation and cataract formation.

CONCLUSIONS

Aspirin acetylates all the lens crystallins as determined by the covalent bonding of ^{14}C acetyl aspirin. 'Cold' aspirin acetylation takes place in the amino groups of all crystallins and prevents the subsequent binding of ^{14}C glucose or ^{14}C prednisone and acetylation by aspirin *in vitro* prevents crystallin oxidation, aggregation and high molecular weight aggregate formation induced by glucose or prednisone. A chemical basis for the protective effect of aspirin in diabetic or steroid cataracts is summarized.

REFERENCES

(1) Cotlier E. Senile cataracts: evidence for acceleration by diabetes and deceleration by salicylate. *Can J Ophthalmol* 1981; **16**: 113–18.
(2) Cotlier E, Sharma YG, Niven T, Brescia M. Distribution of salicylate in lens and intraocular fluids and its effect on cataract formation. *Am J Med* 1983; **74**: 83–90.
(3) Manabe S, Bucala R, Cerami A. Nonenzymatic addition of glucocorticoids to lens proteins in steroid-induced cataracts. *J Clin Invest* 1984; **74**: 1803–10.
(4) Harding JJ. Nonenzymatic covalent posttranslational modification of proteins *in vivo*. *Adv Protein Chem* 1985; **37**: 247–334.
(5) Huby R, Harding JJ. Non-enyzmic glycosylation (glycation) of lens proteins by galactose and protection by aspirin and reduced glutathione. *Exp Eye Res* 1988; **47**: 53–9.
(6) Rao GN, Lardis MP, Cotlier E. Acetylation of lens crystallins: a passive mechanism by which aspirin could prevent cataract formation. *Biochem Biophys Res Commun* 1985; **128**: 1125–32.
(7) Rao GN, Cotlier E. Aspirin prevents the non-enzymatic glycosylation and carbamylation of the human eye lens crystallins *in vitro*. *Biochem Biophys Res Commun* 1988; **151**: 991–6.
(8) Abrahams EC, Swamy MS, Perry RE. *Symposium on the Maillard reaction in aging, diabetes and nutrition*. New York: Alan R Liss Publishers, 1988.
(9) Williams WF, Odon JD. The utilization of ^{13}C and ^{31}P nuclear magnetic resonance spectroscopy in the study of sorbitol pathway and aldose reductase inhibition in intact rabbit lenses. *Exp Eye Res* 1987; **44**: 717–30.
(10) Bucala R, Gallata M, Manabe S, Cotlier E, Cerami A. Glucocorticoid lens protein adducts in experimentally induced steroid cataracts. *Exp Eye Res* 1985; **40**: 853–63.
(11) Urban RC, Cotlier E. Corticosteroid-induced cataracts. *Survey Ophthalm* 1986; **31**: 102–10.

DISCUSSION

Dr Fryers: The effect of ibuprofen and paracetamol found by Dr Harding does not really fit with the acetylation hypothesis, as he acknowledged, but it does seem to fit with Professor Cotlier's figures for the inhibition of the conversion of glucose to sorbitol.

Professor Cotlier: There are still some gaps in trying to marry the basic science with the clinical observations but, if you think in terms of the younger experimental cataracts, you have both non-steroidals and aspirin both of which are inhibitors of the utilization of NADPH. There is a common mechanism.

Dr Harding: Ibuprofen will also decrease the non-enzymic glycosylation just as aspirin does. We have done similar experiments with ibuprofen and it has a very similar effect. It may be that they are binding in another way, but paracetamol does not do that. I have heard it suggested that perhaps a metabolite of paracetamol might bind to proteins and do similar things to the acetylation.

Dr Fryers: Can the lens carry out the metabolism of paracetamol?

Dr Harding: I do not know, nor is it known whether a metabolite would circulate within it.

Dr Fryers: I do not think so; it is too short lived.

Dr Smith: We have been told several times in the last two days that aspirin offers a large first pass effect in the liver; that the de-acetylation takes place there and there is only salicylate circulating. Is there enough acetylsalicylic acid circulating around the eye to acetylate these lens crystallins in the first place?

Dr Fryers: I do not know the answer to the second part, but you are wrong on the first part. If you take aspirin in solution, for instance from effervescent or soluble aspirin, you get quite high but short-lasting levels of aspirin in the general circulation and that is almost certainly the mechanism for the relief of pain, so if it will do one, why should it not do the other? Of course, whether it crosses the barriers to get into the eye would need special study and I am not aware of any having been done.

Professor Cotlier: We undertook some studies, intravenously injecting rabbits with the acetylated form of radioactive aspirin, and we were able to find it in the lens within about 1 minute. We have not done similar tests with orally-administered aspirin, but it does produce *in vivo* acetylation when given intravenously.

Dr Harding: There are other studies by Valeri *et al.* in Rome (1) showing that both aspirin and salicylate reach the lens. In general drugs diffuse into the lens very slowly and diffuse out very slowly so that they accumulate with multiple dosing.

Dr Fryers: In extension of that point, one of the things that I hoped would be discussed is the implication that, if acetylation is the mechanism of action, as the lens protein is there for life, and the acetylation is irreversible, do you have to add aspirin only once? It may be that of each dose only a very small percentage is acetylated so that it may take a long time to get there, but there ought to be some finite length of time or dose level that is needed to get the lens fully acetylated, so that one never need take it again. If that is the case, it would be quite difficult, I imagine, to find adults in the cataract age group who had not during their lives taken enough aspirin to reach that level.

Dr Harding: That is a good point, but the word irreversible implies never changing, and never, in terms of the platelets, is a short time, certainly in contrast to a lens protein. I am not sure that acetylation would be irreversible over 80 years; it may be slowly reversible and the acetyl groups may need replenishing from time to time.

Dr Loose-Wagenbach: Dr Harding, you presented some risk factors. The risk factor for low-dose treatment with aspirin is 0.33. Have you any idea of the relative risk factor if a patient is treated with 100 mg daily for a year?

Dr Harding: We have nobody who has taken 100 mg a day. We are only recording what people have already taken. All I can say is that, as with the heart studies, there is no dose relationship. In every quartile there was a greater proportion of controls taking the drug than the cases, and there was no real difference between the apparent relative risk in each of those quartiles.

Dr Fryers: In low doses you have to remember that the liver first pass take-out of aspirin gets nearer to 100% and it is variable from person to person, so it would really not be possible to predict how much aspirin there would be in the circulation from 100 mg. In some people there would be none.

Professor Cotlier: One has to take into consideration that the process of cataract formation takes place over a period of many years. This is not like pregnancy experiments, which are very short relative to cataract, or platelet circulation, or anticoagulation following a heart attack. Here you are talking about a condition which develops through a period of several years, so the effects of aspirin must take place on an additive and chronic basis, rather than a sort of one-shot or short-term effect. It is more complicated, and I am surprised that we have been able to unravel some of these things so far. There was a point at which it did not appear we could get any idea of how aspirin was working. You must remember that aspirin has to go around the general circulation into the aqueous humour, from the aqueous humour into the lens itself, and so on, so there are many steps through which a drug has to go in order to be effective in the tissue, and that is why there are still quite a few unanswered questions. However, I am satisfied that we have answered some of the major ones.

Dr Fryers: Diabetics age and deteriorate more quickly than the rest of the population. Presumably the property you are describing as regards lens protein is fairly common, because most of the proteins that have been studied glycate, and some of these proteins must be rather critical. Obviously, enzymes, and similar substances, may not be replaced very quickly and in some people there may also be a relative deficiency of an enzyme production mechanism so that glycating it will render it less effective. Thus, it is just like ageing, with less and less ability, and that is the sort of thing that happens in diabetics; they seem to go through all the processes of ageing a little faster than non-diabetics.

Dr Harding: Cerami (2) has suggested that non-enzymic glycosylation is an important mechanism in ageing. I would extend that and say: not just non-enzymic glycosylation but other reactions, such as those with cyanate, steroids and acetaldehyde could cause age-related damage (3). These (molecules) all attack proteins. The nuclear lens proteins are in an unfortunate position in that they are never renewed but there are other proteins that are renewed fairly slowly, like collagen in the basement membranes, that are affected in diabetes. There are myelin proteins and it is to me not perhaps a coincidence that peripheral neuropathy is found not only in diabetes but also in renal failure, and was found in cyanate therapy when it was given for sickle cell disease. All these things are associated with non-enzymic modification of proteins. Now we find that aspirin is able to prevent some of these non-enzymic modifications, and that could have interesting implications.

REFERENCES

(1) Valeri P, Romanelli L, de Paolis L, Martinelli B. Ocular distribution of aspirin and salicylate following systemic administration of aspirin to rabbits. *J Pharm Pharmacol* 1988; **40**: 823–24.
(2) Cerami A, Vlassara H, Brownlee M. Glucose and aging. *Sci Am* 1987; **256**: 90–6.
(3) Harding JJ, Beswick HT, Ajiboye R, Huby R, Blakytny R, Ruxon KC. Non-enzymic post-translational modification of proteins in aging. A review. *Mech Ageing Dev* 1989; **50**: 7–16.